MUSCLE

Jason Maxwell

Legal Disclaimer

Warning: All the information presented in *Muscle* is for educational and resource purposes only. It is not a substitute for or in addition to any advice given to you by your physician or health care provider.

Consult your physician before making any changes to your lifestyle, diet, or exercise habits. You are solely responsible for the way information in *Muscle* is perceived and utilized and so, you do so at your own risk.

In no way will Jason Maxwell or Jason Maxwell Consulting Ltd, or any persons associated with *Muscle* be held responsible for any injuries or problems that may occur due to the use of this book or the advice contained within.

Personal Disclaimer

We are not doctors, nor do we possess a degree in nutrition. The advice we give is based on years of practical application, dealing with the needs of our own health and physiques as well as the needs of others. Any recommendations we may make to you regarding diet or exercise, including supplements and herbal or nutritional treatments must be discussed between you and your doctor(s).

Muscle-Building Disclaimer

Required Legal Disclaimer: Due to recent laws from the FTC, it is required that all companies identify what a "typical" result is. The truth is that most people never do anything when it comes to trying building muscle. They might buy a million products, including this one, but never do anything with the information they have in hand. The testimonials that you saw were of people who took action, followed a healthy lifestyle, exercised, and ate a balanced nutritional diet. If you want results like them, you should do this too.

Copyright Notice

For my 18-year-old self,

Skinny-Fat Jason Maxwell,

Who had zero confidence and didn't know what he was doing in an empty gym. When Elon Musk invents the time machine, I'll send you a copy in a DeLorean.

Don't worry, I've got your back.

Table of Contents

SECTION 1:
THE STUPID SIMPLE SOLUTION

Chapter 1:
Muscle: How I Gained 27 Pounds of Muscle in Four Months and How You Can Too

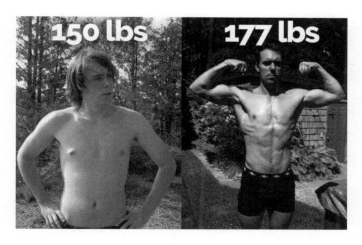

It was a hot, humid summer when I started lifting. And I didn't know what in hell I was doing.

I walked into an empty gym and looked around. Even with zero people there, I was intimidated. Dumbbells, bars, plates, and machines: a bodybuilder's paradise. And I was a deer in the headlights.

I wanted to get jacked. I wanted a six-pack. I wanted a body that could get me a high school sweetheart. So I did what any other beginner would do. I ran on the treadmill for 30 minutes and did some sit-ups and biceps curls.

I was about 17, and I was fed up with being trapped in an ugly body. I was skinny-fat and had zero confidence. I was sick of being single and of not having the courage even to talk to a girl. Why would a girl talk to me? I had a terrible body.

I remember going to high school parties, getting drunk, and trying to talk to the girls I had crushes on. They wanted nothing to do with me. Rejection. Rejection. Rejection.

I was so embarrassed of my body that I wore baggy clothes. I was hiding my body, while the high school jocks showed off their physiques and dated the girls I liked.

I had this one friend, Andy, and I was always envious of his body. I remember thinking to myself, "if I could just build a body like Andy, then I'd be happy." Andy had what I wanted: a six-pack, wide shoulders, biceps with veins that popped. I was super jealous.

I kept lifting throughout high school and made a bit of progress on a bro split routine. I gained a small amount of muscle and lost a little fat, but I still didn't look the way I wanted to. I wanted to be jacked. I wanted to look like a superhero. I thought "well, I'm doing the work, and nothing's happening, so it's obviously my genetics. I'm doomed forever."

Thankfully, I did a bit of research and discovered that bro splits don't work well for beginners. I learned, moreover, that if you really want to build muscle, you need to do something else.

That "something else" changed my life! And in this book I'll reveal what that "something else" is for your benefit.

When I was 19 and on my way to university, I told myself, "I'm going to do everything right. I'm going to do what's supposed to work for guys like me, and I'm going to track my macros: calories, carbs, proteins, and fats. If I don't gain muscle, then I'll know it's my genetics."

I weighed 150 lb. (68 kg) when I left home for university at the end of August. A few months later, I returned for Christmas break a toned 177 lb. (80 kg). I walked in the door, and my brother took one look at me and said, "holy shit…your neck is huge!"

My fitness journey was under way.

Over the next few years, I experimented with different fitness techniques as I pursued my aerospace engineering degree at Ryerson University, in Toronto, Canada. Yes, I'm literally a rocket scientist, and it had long been my intention to become an astronaut. But as I got more into fitness, I realized that my passion was helping guys build muscle.

I graduated top three in my class and never looked back. The day after graduating, I was working as a personal trainer in Toronto, making $16 an hour, with a $30,000 student loan to pay off. It made no sense financially, but I was following my heart.

In the decade since, I've tried numerous approaches to and read everything I could about building muscle. I've distilled what I've learned into this book.

Whether you're a beginner, an intermediate, or an advanced trainee, this book will help you achieve fantastic results. This is the book I wish I'd had when I started training. If I'd known then what I know now, I'd probably be 15 lb. (7 kg) heavier and stronger.

This book introduces you to methods that have always worked to get people jacked. They worked in the 1800s. They worked in the 1900s. They work now. This is the timeless approach to building muscle, and I'm happy to have you here. Welcome to *Muscle*.

Chapter 2:
To Men Who Want to Build 27 Pounds of Muscle in Three Months

I'll never forget the day I started doing things right. I was 19 years old, and I was moving from my small Canadian hometown, population 3,500, to Toronto, a city of 2.5 million people. Little did I know that this would be among the best decisions I'd ever make.

I was a skinny-fat 150 lb. (68 kg), 5'11" (1.8 m) teenager. I hated the way I looked. What I saw in the mirror didn't reflect masculinity. Staring back at me was a two-pack of abs, narrow shoulders, and wide hips. I blamed this on poor genetics. The guys on such reality TV shows as *Survivor*, *Big Brother*, and *The Bachelor* (don't judge) were jacked. I assumed you had to be born that way and there was nothing you could do otherwise. Was I wrong!

I moved into my university dorm and a small room with cinder block walls and a full kitchen. The campus also had a state-of-the-art gym. This meant I could do my best to change my body. I could cook for myself and work out.

I had no idea what I was doing and just ballparked everything. I ate 3,000 calories a day because that sounded like a good number and divided my intake into 33% carbs, 34% protein, and 33% fat. I did full-body workouts three to four times a week with my training partner, Marc. He was a great guy, and we'd encourage each other to lift heavier and heavier loads. I just felt that if I ate that many calories a day and trained that many times a week using big combination lifts I'd be able to at least improve my body. I had no idea how effective this program would be.

Fast-forward three months. I went home for Christmas weighing 177 lb. (80 kg). I walked through the door of my house, and my brother exclaimed, "holy shit!" I'll never forget that. I asked him, "what?" and he said, "your neck is huge, and you're looking bigger."

That night, I went out with friends, and the next day one of them told me that everyone was talking about how much bigger I'd gotten. They'd noticed that my neck, arms, shoulders, back, and legs had all grown. This made sense given that in just three months I'd gained 27 lb. (12 kg) and, crazy as it sounds, completely changed my body. I had a six-pack. My shoulders were wide and my waist narrow. I'd also lost fat, which means that I'd gained more than the 27 lb. of muscle the scale indicated I'd packed on my frame.

Gaining 27 lb. of muscle without drugs in only three months might seem ridiculous, but I know it's possible. I did it, and I've seen my clients do it time and time again. This is what broscientists call newbie gains. If someone who hasn't worked out much starts training hard and correctly, the magic will happen. The body will gain a bunch of muscle in the first year of training and then become harder and harder every year after that. This is demonstrated by muscle scholar Lyle McDonald's Natural Lean Muscle Mass Gain Model.

Years Training	Muscle Gain (lb.)
1	20–25 (9–11 kg)
2	10–12 (4.5–5.5 kg)
3	5–6 (2–3 kg)
4	2–3 (1–1.5 kg)

This model is consistent with my experience, of my gains and of my clients'. If you're a newbie, you will gain the most muscle in the first couple months of your first training year. Gains are not linear.

Another model that I like is Alan Aragon's Natural Lean Muscle Mass Gain Model.

Category	Years Training	Muscle Gain
Beginner	1 year or less	1–1.5% total body weight per month
Intermediate	2–3 years	0.5–1% total body weight per month
Advanced	5 years or more	0.25–0.5% total body weight per month

Aragon's model suggests that I should have gained 2.3 lb. (1 kg) of muscle per month and a maximum of 27.9 lbs (13 kg) for the full year. In fact, I gained pretty much all of that in just my first three months of training. Over the next nine months, I didn't gain much muscle. It wasn't until the second year when I started gaining muscle again.

My anomalies aside, I encourage you to refer to this chapter and the models presented above for an idea of how much muscle you can expect to gain year by year. It'll help you with realistic expectations. If, for instance, you weight 150 lb. (68 kg), don't expect to gain 80 lb. (36 kg) of muscle your first year of training.

What's the Most Muscle I Can Gain throughout My Lifetime, Drug Free?

This is an interesting question, and research shows that you can get a pretty accurate answer. It's fun to figure out how much muscle you can gain in your lifetime, known as your maximum muscular potential. It's no different than going to the doctor when you're four years old and having the doctor predict that you'll be 6' tall. Many times the doctor is right, but sometimes the estimate can be off by as much as 5–10%. The same holds true with the following formula.

The formula to finding your maximum muscular potential is based on your fat free mass index (FFMI), which, in a nutshell, is a number corresponding to your height, weight, and body fat percentage. Research shows that a natural, drug-free FFMI corresponds to an upper limit of approximately 25. In other words, an all-natural body has an FFMI of 25 or less. Now, remember that 25 is an approximate number. I've met natural guys with an FFMI of almost 27. The key is that there is probably a margin for error of about 10%. Your FFMI could range between 23 and 27.

Knowing your FFMI is interesting, but it's better to know how much muscle mass you can gain: your maximum lean mass (MLM) potential. So I've extrapolated the following formula from the FFMI:

$$MLM = 25*(Height^2)$$

In this case, your height is measured in meters, and your MLM is measured in kilograms. So let's say that you are 6' (1.8 m) tall. This is how to calculate your MLM:

MLM = 25*(1.83 meters)^2 = 25/3.35 = 83.7 kg of lean mass

If at 83.7 kg of lean mass you are 10% body fat, you weigh 93 kg, or 205 lb. That's lean and jacked and natural.

That is your maximum genetic potential. Obviously, there will still be some variance, but this gives you a good starting point. Only you know if you are truly natural, so who cares what anyone else says? Aim for the maximum genetic potential using this formula, and if you surpass it naturally, that's awesome. But at least you had a clear quantitative goal in mind from the outset.

Reference

Obadike, Obi. "Ask The Ripped Dude: ''How Much Muscle Can I Put On Naturally?''. "*Bodybuilding.com*, 9 Nov. 2015, www.bodybuilding.com/fun/ask-the-ripped-dude-how-much-muscle-can-i-put-on-naturally.html.

Chapter 3:
Steve Reeves's Secret to Head-on Collisions

The late Steve Reeves arguably had the best physique in bodybuilding. It turned heads and caused at least one head-on collision.

In the late 1950s, Reeves was posing for a photo shoot in his bikini bottoms alongside a highway in Southern California. His body gleamed under the sun as beads of sweat ran down his pumped up his muscles while he held a double biceps pose to perfection.

Everyone in the cars driving by rolled down their windows for a glimpse of this modern-day Hercules. Suddenly, a car blasted through the traffic barrier, narrowly missing Steve and the photographer before hurtling downhill and crashing head-on into a tree.

Now, I know what you're thinking—that Reeves sprinted down the hill, muscles rippling with every leap and bound, and tore through twisted metal with his bare hands to save the driver. But that's not what happened.

Reeves and the photographer stared at the car in shock. After all, they'd almost been killed. As smoke and steam arose from the engine, the driver opened his door and walked out, unharmed. He approached Steve and told him, "You have the greatest body man has ever seen. I couldn't stop looking as I drove by, and now look at what happened!" Months later, Steve was cast in the lead role in the movie *Hercules*.

Reeves had a secret to building his body: proportions. He believed that his body was akin to a raw piece of marble and that if he could sculpt it in the pattern of a Greek god or of a masterwork by Da Vinci or Michelangelo he would look fantastic. He understood that there are certain ratios on the male body that people find incredibly attractive.

Among these is the so-called Golden Ratio. It suggests that the ideal waist to shoulder ratio for a lean male is 1:1.618. When you divide your shoulder circumference by your waist circumference, you want the number to be as near 1.618 as possible. Achieving this ratio requires that you increase the size of your shoulders, trim your waist, or both. When you get as close as possible to the 1:1.618 ratio, your body will look more muscular even if you haven't gained muscle.

Reeves also believed that for perfect symmetry, your arms, calves, and neck needed to be the same size. He felt, moreover, that your arms should be 252% of your wrist circumference and that your waist should be 86% and your chest 148%, respectively, of the circumference of your pelvis as measured around that part of your hips where you wear your pants.

Using Reeves's measurements, we are able to reverse engineer and better see the ideal proportions of the male body.

- Arms: 18.5 inches (47 cm)
- Calves: 18.5 inches (47 cm)
- Neck: 18.5 inches (47 cm)
- Forearms: 14.75 inches (38 cm)
- Thighs: 27 inches (69 cm)
- Waist: 30 inches (76 cm)
- Chest: 54 inches (137 cm)
- Height: 6 feet 1 inch (186 cm)

I've created the following table to show the proportions that Reeves sought:

Body Part	Measurement
Arms	2.52 x wrist size
Calves	2.52 x wrist size
Neck	2.52 x wrist size
Thighs	1.46 x calf size
Waist	0.86 x pelvis circumference size (measured where you wear your pants) or waist size when lean
Chest	1.48 x pelvis size (measured where you wear your pants) or 1.72 x waist size
Shoulders	1.618 x waist size
Forearms	0.8 x arm size

Using these proportions, let's figure out your ideal measurements.

Measure your wrist at its smallest diameter. My wrist, for example, is 17 cm (7 inches) in circumference. This measurement enables me to determine my arm, calf, and neck sizes:

Arm size = 2.52 x wrist size = 2.52 x 17 cm = 42.8 cm

My arms, calves, and neck should each be about 42.8 cm at their largest diameter. And, from the table above, we know that my thighs should be 1.46 x my calf circumference:

Thigh size = 1.46 x calf size = 1.46 x 42.8 = 62.5 cm

We also know that my forearms, measured at their largest diameter, should be 0.8 x my arm circumference:

Forearm size = 0.8 x arm size = 34.2 cm

My waist, according the table above, should be about 0.86 x my pelvis circumference. This measurement needs to be taken when you are lean, with a body fat percentage below 12%. Rather than measuring the pelvis, you can simply measure your waist at its smallest diameter when you are at your leanest, below 12% body fat. My waist is about 76 cm.

With my lean waist size, I can determine my shoulder size using the Golden Ratio:

Shoulder size = 1.618 x waist size = 1.618 x 76 cm = 123 cm

I can also determine my chest size using my lean waist size:

Chest size = 1.72 x waist size = 1.72 x 76 cm = 130.7 cm

So my final ideal measurements are as follows:

Body Part	Measurement
Arms	42.8 cm (17 inches)
Calves	42.8 cm (17 inches)
Neck	42.8 cm (17 inches)
Thighs	62.5 cm (25 inches)
Waist	76 cm (30 inches)
Chest	130.7 cm (52 inches)
Shoulders	123 cm (48 inches)
Forearms	34.2 cm (14 inches)

It's great to know our ideal measurements. The question is, how do we attain them? I'll give you the exact game plan later in this book. For now, suffice it to say that you will achieve your ideal measurements in the specialization phase of the *Muscle* program. I've made this handy chart to determine where, depending on your measurements, you will need to specialize.

Measurement	What to Specialize
Arms	Biceps and triceps
Calves	Calves
Neck	Neck
Thighs	Quadriceps and hamstrings
Waist	Fat loss
Chest	Pectorals and back muscles
Shoulders	Lateral, medial, and rear deltoids
Forearms	Forearm

When you train your body, your goal should not be to just get as big as possible. You should also strive to build an aesthetically pleasing body. Measurements will help you get there. After all, you lift weights to look and feel good. You do not lift weights to become a troll or caveman.

Reference

Robson, David. "Know Your Measurements For Bodybuilding Success." *Bodybuilding.com*, 18 Mar. 2015, www.bodybuilding.com/fun/drobson207.htm.

Chapter 4
Five Methods to Build Muscle Quickly by Analyzing the Muscle Curve

The most successful muscle-building programs need to be analyzed for what works and then improved upon. Almost everything is subjected to this process. Take the airplane, for example. I know from my background in aerospace engineering that the first thing you do before designing an airplane is to benchmark what is already successful. You take the best-performing aircraft for the task at hand, reverse engineer it, and then improve upon its design.

Tim Ferriss states in his book *The 4-Hour Body* that you can learn the most from the extremes of the bell curve. For Ferris, this means analyzing what works for professional bodybuilders and what works with patients rehabilitating injuries that resulted in large muscle loss. This makes perfect sense, but I don't think Ferriss's model directly applies to people reading this book. You're here because you want to build muscle, look incredible, and feel fantastic.

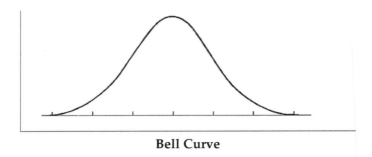

Bell Curve

Ferriss's model needs to be adjusted for people who want to build muscle, look incredible, and feel fantastic. It needs to target an end result and furnish only relevant muscle-building knowledge. The only extremes we need to analyze are drug-using and drug-free bodybuilders. The middle of the curve, then, represents everyone else who trains to build muscle. All the guys bench pressing at the gym represent the middle of the curve. Ignore them and focus on the training methods of drug-using and drug-free pro bodybuilders.

Go a step further and compare two groups of bodybuilders: modern and golden age. The goals of bodybuilding have changed over the past few decades. In the golden age, the goal was symmetry first and size second. In modern times, it's vice versa. I said in the previous chapter that your goal should be to build muscle and a well-proportioned body. This is why I like to compare these two groups of bodybuilders. What can we learn from them? My research and experience reveals five main themes.

Get strong.

Bodybuilders are strong. Golden age bodybuilder Tom Platz was known for his strong and large legs. They were gigantic compared with the rest of his body. His secret? Squatting heavy weights for lots of reps. You are probably picturing 225–315 lb. (102–143 kg). After all, that is pretty heavy. But no, Tom Platz would squat 525 lb. (238 kg) for 23 reps. Yes, he was drug assisted, but you can't deny that he was strong.

Many modern bodybuilders have backgrounds in powerlifting. Take drug-free competitor Dr. Layne Norton. He's a pro bodybuilder with a foundation of strength. As of this writing, he holds a squat record of 303 kg (668 lbs) and a deadlift record of 322.5 kg (711 lbs).

Build muscle in the gym and control body weight with diet.

We've all done this, wake up one morning and say, I'm going to lose weight. What's the first thing we do? Focus on cardio by switching to light weights and high reps. This is not how to lose fat. Bodybuilders, past and present, lift weights to build or maintain muscle. They regulate their body weight with diet.

Building muscle means more food. Losing fat means less food.

Use high weekly training volumes.

Simply defined, volume is the number of total reps for an exercise. High volume indicates high numbers of reps each week and usually leads to big, strong muscles.

A look at golden age bodybuilding programs, such as Steve Reeves's full-body program, reveals high weekly training volumes. Reeves trained each body part with 3–4 sets of 8–15 reps daily. This isn't a huge daily volume, but Reeves did his full-body routine three days a week. So he was doing 9–12 sets of 8–15 reps for each body part weekly. This quickly adds up.

If a muscle is lagging, build it up.

Think of your body as a block of marble. You are the sculptor and have the ability to shape your proportions to your satisfaction. Your body is your masterpiece. Desire large arms or shoulders? Specialize on them. This is what bodybuilders have always done and continue to do.

Feel the muscle working.

When you train a muscle, you want it to contract as hard as possible. This requires actively thinking about and feeling the muscle working. Before executing a biceps curl, for instance, make a fist and pretend to curl. Flex your biceps hard. When you can do this, curl with weight. You will be able to put massive tension on and signal to the body to make the muscle grow.

Reference

Wolff-Mann, Ethan. "How Much Could Arnold Schwarzenegger Really Lift?" *Thrillist*, Thrillist, 17 Dec. 2014, www.thrillist.com/gear/how-strong-was-arnold-schwarzenegger-at-weight-lifting.

Chapter 5:
Three Proven Muscle Growth Mechanisms

A fundamental understanding of what causes a muscle to grow is important. And that's exactly what a research paper written in 2010 by muscle scientist Brad Schoenfeld provides. Dr. Schoenfeld found that there are three mechanisms responsible for muscle growth: mechanical tension, metabolic stress, and muscle damage.

Mechanical Tension

Imagine a tug-of-war: two teams pulling on a rope in opposite directions as hard as they can. The rope gets increasingly taut. Cut in the middle, it would snap like an elastic. This is tension, and it occurs in your muscles when you lift a weight, flex, or even stretch under load.

That tension disturbs muscle integrity and elicits molecular and cellular responses that tell the muscle to grow bigger, stronger. To build muscle, you need to feel it contract. Then you'll know that you're putting it under adequate tension to effect growth.

Metabolic Stress

You'll know metabolic stress when it occurs. It's that pumped, burning sensation you get amid extreme exertion and that results from a buildup of metabolites in the muscle, including lactate, hydrogen ions, inorganic phosphate, and creatine. Though unpleasant, it's vital to muscle growth, and I've found the best way to cause metabolic stress is through high rep exercises, drop sets, rest pauses, and partials. These all pump up and make muscle burn.

Muscle Damage

You know the running joke about leg day. You train your legs, and the next day you can't take stairs, can't sit on the toilet, and can barely walk. It's funnier on paper than in real life. The pain indicates that you've damaged muscle, but this unpleasantness, too, is a crucial, third mechanism to building muscle.

You've probably heard that you need to break muscle down so it can rebuild bigger and stronger. Although there is some truth in this, it's not exactly what happens. What does happen when you train hard is damage muscle fibers such that they become inflamed and cause you pain perhaps a few days after training. This inflammatory response releases growth factors in the body that regulate muscle growth. I've found that damaging muscle to induce the release of growth factors is best achieved through high volume (lots of repetitions); loaded stretching, which also causes mechanical tension; and an emphasis on the eccentric (lowering with gravity) portion of a lift.

Putting It All Together

You build muscle through the three mechanisms of mechanical tension, metabolic stress, and muscle damage, and they are not necessarily mutually exclusive. You don't have to train for mechanical tension one day, metabolic stress the next day, and muscle damage the day after that. All three can be combined in a single, full workout.

Any time you lift a weight, mechanical tension is present. The more weight the greater the tension, but there is always tension. It's just the way it works. Metabolic stress occurs when you lift close to failure. Muscle damage can happen on any lift, and especially on a lift you're not accustomed to. Building muscle with these mechanisms requires the following:

1. A focus on feeling the muscle contracting.
2. An occasional pumped-up feeling in the muscle.
3. Muscle soreness sometimes up to 48 hours after a workout.

Reference

Contreras, Bret. "The Hypertrophy Specialist." *T NATION*, 27 Oct. 2010, www.t-nation.com/training/hypertrophy-specialist.

Chapter 6:
The 80/20 Rule and the Muscle Pyramid

To get the best results, you must focus on what works best. According to the 80/20 rule, 80% of your best results come from 20% of what you do. Following this rule is highly effective in all aspects of life, including building muscle.

Focusing on the 20% of what works best in your training will give you 80% of your muscle-building gains faster and more effectively than possible otherwise. What works best? It comes down to following what I call the muscle pyramid.

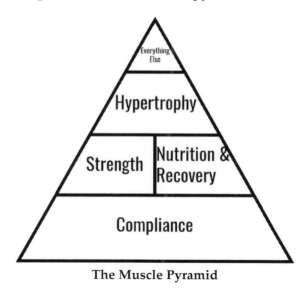

The Muscle Pyramid

The pyramid consists of five sections from its base up: compliance, strength, nutrition and recovery, hypertrophy, and everything else.

Compliance

Meet Tom and Steve. Tom has an excellent muscle-building program. Done correctly, it will add 1 lb. (0.5 kg) of muscle per week. Tom's goal is to gain 10 lb. (4.5 kg) of muscle, so he needs to do his program for 10 weeks straight. Steve found an inferior program on the Internet. It will add 1 lb. of muscle a month, done correctly. Steve's goal is also 10 lb. of muscle. But he needs to do his program for 10 consecutive months.

Who will build muscle fastest? Logic suggests Tom. The fact is, however, it depends on how they do their programs. If Tom skips workouts, substitutes exercises on a whim, and follows his program only 20% of the time, he'll impair his ability to gain 1 lb. of muscle per week. With 20% program compliance, Tom can expect results of 20%, if he's lucky. If Steve, on the other hand, is 100% compliant with his program, he'll gain the desired 10 lb. of muscle in 10 months.

Compliance thus is the base of the pyramid, because compliance leads to results. As with Steve's and Tom's examples, an inferior program followed faithfully could achieve results superior to the best program in the world if your compliance with the latter sucks.

Strength

Moving up the pyramid, we come to strength, the ability to lift ever-heavier weights. Tom goes to the gym and murders his muscles. He lifts light weights and only chases the pump. Steve, conversely, strives every workout for one more rep or at least 5 lb. more than last workout.

Who will build more muscle? In the short term, it'll be Tom. But month after month, Steve will get stronger and build more muscle than Tom. Strength is fundamental to muscle acquisition. If Tom can bench press 135 lb. (61 kg) for 10 reps and Steve can bench press 225 lb. (102 kg) for 10 reps, Steve obviously will have stronger and bigger pecs. Building muscle calls for lifting increasingly heavy weights, and that, in turn, requires strength. It's as simple as that.

Many guys go into the gym thinking they don't need to get stronger or to power lift. This mentality robs them of muscle gains. Many professional bodybuilders were once or are also powerlifters. One of them you may have heard of, Arnold Schwarzenegger.

As a teenager, Schwarzenegger learned power and Olympic lifts. At only 17, he won his first weight-lifting competition. He defended that title the next year and then went on to win two powerlifting competitions, at ages 19 and 21. This was before his inaugural Mr. Olympia contest. The Austrian Oak's physique was built on strength. His personal records are as follows:

- Clean and press, 264 lbs (120 kg)
- Snatch, 243 lbs (110 kg)
- Clean and jerk, 298 lbs (135 kg)
- Squat, 545 lbs (247 kg)
- Bench press, 520 lbs (236 kg)
- Deadlift, 710 lbs (322 kg)

Nutrition and Recovery

Nutrition and recovery equal strength in importance on the muscle pyramid, something Tom fails to grasp. He stays up late playing video games. He then wakes early and buys a double espresso to kickstart his day. The rest of the day he eats fast food and drinks coffee to stay awake. When he goes to the gym, he takes a pre-workout supplement to boost his energy. He seldom feels vigorous enough to complete workouts and afterwards is sore for over a week. Four to five nights a week, he drinks with friends and eats copious amounts of bar food.

Will Tom build a lot of muscle? Probably not. His recovery and nutrition suck. Steve, on the other hand, gets eight hours of sleep nightly, eats lots of meat and vegetables, and has amazing energy for his workouts. Steve is doing things right.

Hypertrophy

Earlier, I said that Tom will build muscle from constantly pumping and demolishing his muscle. You know now that muscle is built through mechanical tension, metabolic stress, and muscle damage. Strength work handles most of the mechanical tension, but it's hypertrophy work that involves all three mechanisms for building muscles. Strength enables you to lift more when you start to focus on the high-volume hypertrophy work that leads to the sensation of pumped-up muscles and to muscle soreness lasting, possibly, for up to five days and hopefully no more.

Everything Else

The "everything else" section of the muscle pyramid involves injury prevention, tempo, rest periods, and exercise selection. This is the least important of the pyramid's components and should take up less than 20% of your time.

Reference

"Arnold Schwarzenegger." *Wikipedia*, Wikimedia Foundation, 26 Mar. 2018, en.wikipedia.org/wiki/Arnold_Schwarzenegger.

Chapter 7:
How Strong Is Strong Enough?

Hopefully, you by now accept that building muscle requires strength and that strength is the foundation to everything you do in the gym. The question is, "how strong is strong enough?" That's the heavy subject this chapter hopes to shed light on.

The 300/400/500 Club

In 1991, Stuart McRobert wrote in his book *Brawn* that a lean, adult man who could bench press 300 lb. (136 kg), squat 400 lb. (181 kg), and deadlift 500 lb. (227 kg) would have a fantastic physique. With strength, MrcRobert maintained, muscle will follow.

Have you ever seen someone with less than 15% body fat who bench presses 300 lb., squats 400 lb., and deadlifts 500 lb.? You'd know them for a broad chest, wide shoulders, thick back, and big, meaty legs. That said, however, McRobert's is a sort of one-size-fits-all strategy. What if injury prevents you from squatting, deadlifting, or bench pressing? Adjustments are needed.

We need first to have strength standards for chest, back, shoulders, and legs. Second, we need bilateral and unilateral variations, two limbs vs one, in other words. Third, we need two categories of strength: strong and aesthetically strong, the equivalent of the 300/400/500 club.

The numbers I'm about to provide are from the 300/400/500 club but are based on strength for a 200 lb. (91 kg) person with below 15% body fat. This is important because strength should be calculated relative to body weight. A high body weight increases your chances of being strong. Of course, looking heavy outside the gym instead of looking as if you lift heavy is not desirable. As my friend Gregory O'Gallagher from Kinobody says, "fat doesn't lift weight. Muscles do."

Chest Strength Standards

- **Strong:** Bench press = 1.25 x body weight for 1 repetition
- **Aesthetically strong:** Bench press = 1.5 x body weight for 1 repetition

Body Weight (lbs)	Strong Bench Press 1 Rep Max (lb.)	Aesthetically Strong Bench Press 1 Rep Max (lb.)
150	187.5	225
175	218.75	262.5
200	250	300
225	281.25	337.5

- **Strong:** Single-arm dumbbell bench press = 0.5 x body weight for 1 repetition
- **Aesthetically Strong:** Single-arm dumbbell bench press = 0.6 x body weight for 1 repetition

Body Weight (lb.)	Strong Single-Arm Bench Press 1 Rep Max (lb.)	Aesthetically Strong Single-Arm Bench Press 1 Rep Max (lb.)
150	75	90
175	87.5	105
200	100	120
225	112.5	135

Back Strength Standards

- **Strong:** Weighted chin-up = 0.6 x body weight for 1 repetition
- **Aesthetically Strong:** Weighted chin-up = 0.75 x body weight for 1 repetition

Body Weight (lb.)	Strong Weighted Chin-up 1 Rep Max (lb.)	Aesthetically Strong Weighted Chin-up 1 Rep Max (lb.)
150	90	112.5
175	105	131.25
200	120	150
225	135	168.75

Note: I don't give a strength standard for single-arm chin-ups (the unilateral exercise) because most people can't do even 1 body weight repetition.

Shoulder Strength Standards

- **Strong:** Barbell military press = 0.8 x body weight for 1 repetition
- **Aesthetically Strong:** Barbell military press = 1 x body weight for 1 repetition

Body Weight (lb.)	Strong Barbell Military Press 1 Rep Max (lb.)	Aesthetically Strong Barbell Military Press 1 Rep Max (lb.)
150	120	150
175	140	175
200	160	200
225	180	225

- **Strong:** Single-arm dumbbell military press = 0.333 x body weight for 1 repetition
- **Aesthetically Strong:** Single-arm dumbbell military press = 0.4 x body weight for 1 repetition

Body Weight (lb.)	Strong Single-Arm Dumbbell Military Press 1 Rep Max (lb.)	Aesthetically Strong Single-Arm Dumbbell Military Press 1 Rep Max (lb.)
150	50	60
175	58.33	70
200	66.67	80
225	75	90

Leg Strength Standards

Knee-Dominant Exercises

- **Strong:** Back squat = 1.65 x body weight for 1 repetition
- **Aesthetically Strong:** Back squat = 2 x body weight for 1 repetition

Body Weight (lb.)	Strong Back Squat 1 Rep Max (lb.)	Aesthetically Strong Back Squat 1 Rep Max (lb.)
150	247.5	300
175	288.75	350
200	330	400
225	371.25	350

- **Strong:** Bulgarian split squat = 1 x body weight for 1 repetition
- **Aesthetically Strong:** Bulgarian split squat = 1.2 x body weight for 1 repetition

Body Weight (lb.)	Strong Bulgarian Split Squat 1 Rep Max (lb.)	Aesthetically Strong Bulgarian Split Squat 1 Rep Max (lb.)
150	150	180
175	175	210
200	200	240
225	225	270

Hip-Dominant Exercises

- **Strong:** Deadlift = 2 x body weight for 1 repetition

- **Aesthetically Strong:** Deadlift = 2.5 x body weight for 1 repetition

Body Weight (lb.)	Strong Deadlift 1 Rep Max (lb.)	Aesthetically Strong Deadlift 1 Rep Max (lb.)
150	300	375
175	350	437.5
200	400	500
225	350	562.5

- **Strong:** Single-leg deadlift = 1.35 x body weight for 1 repetition
- **Aesthetically Strong:** Single-leg deadlift = 1.65 x body weight for 1 repetition

Body Weight (lb.)	Strong Bulgarian Split Squat 1 Rep Max (lb.)	Aesthetically Strong Bulgarian Split Squat 1 Rep Max (lb.)
150	202.5	247.5
175	236.25	288.75
200	270	330
225	303.75	371.25

Testing Your Lifts

These strength standards are great. But which should you strive for, and how do you test them? I recommend picking one exercise each to test for chest, back, and shoulder strength. For legs, pick one knee-dominant and one hip-dominant exercise.

I have back issues, so I stick to unilateral exercises for my upper body and to Bulgarian split squat and single-leg deadlifts for my legs. For my upper body, where I have no problems other than my back, I do bench press, barbell military press, and chin-ups. Someone with problematic shoulders should stick to unilateral upper-body exercises and do bilateral lower-body work. Guys with no injuries or pains should go with all bilateral exercises. It'll make the process easier. Anyone with pain, meanwhile, is advised to see a doctor and physiotherapist. Pain is not good.

After you've selected your exercises, test one per day to ensure that you are fresh to accurately determine strength. I recommend testing your one repetition max (1RM) once every 6–12 months. In my case, I'd test the bench press on Monday, chin-ups on Tuesday, barbell military press on Wednesday, Bulgarian split squat on Thursday, and single-leg deadlifts on Friday. Each day, apply the following protocol to determine your strength in each lift:

1. Pick a light weight and do the exercise for 5 reps (5 reps on each limb if you're using a unilateral exercise).
2. Rest 3–5 minutes.
3. Add 5–10 lb. (2.3–4.5 kg) and do the exercise again for 5 reps.
4. Rest 3–5 minutes.

5. Repeat steps 3 and 4 until you get to a weight that feels heavy for 5 reps.
6. Add 5 lb. and do the exercise again for 4 reps.
7. Rest 3–5 minutes.
8. Add 5 lb. and do the exercise again for 3 reps.
9. Rest 3–5 minutes.
10. Add 5 lb. and do the exercise again for 2 reps.
11. Rest 3–5 minutes.
12. Add 5 lb. and do the exercise again for 1 rep.
13. Rest 3–5 minutes.
14. Repeat steps 12 and 13 until you cannot lift the weight. Record the last lifted weight; it's your 1RM for that specific exercise.

Reference

McRobert, Stuart. *Brawn: Bodybuilding for the Drug-free and Genetically Typical*. Nicosia, Cyprus: CS Pub., 2007.

Chapter 8:
Use Pain to Your Advantage

The formula to success in all things is the motivation to change something. You obviously are motivated improve your body by building muscle. What's the cause of this motivation? Were you bullied? Do you lack confidence? Do you want to be a role model for your children?

Pain is a powerful motivator. We'll often do whatever it takes to eliminate such pain. Harness it, and you'll find your motivation. If you can't come up with a good pain motivator naturally, create one. Tell a friend, for example, that you'll give him or her X amount of money if you don't build X amount of muscle in 12 months. Your friend will hold you to it, and you'll have the motivation you need to succeed on pain of losing money.

With your motivation in place, you'll need to define an outcome goal: "I want to build X amount of muscle in X amount of time." That's a clear outcome with a clear time period. Establishing a term for achieving an outcome is a vital motivator. Many people fail to achieve outcome goals because they fail to set deadlines. Open-ended goals provide no motivation to act with vigor.

Use the lifting standards and body part measurements in previous chapters to help you set an outcome goal. Aim, for instance, to reach your maximum muscular potential and build ideal proportions. Then define a realistic time period for accomplishing your outcome goal.

Next, set behavior goals—small steps toward achieving your outcome goal. Your behavior goals should ensure compliance with your muscle-building program and include committing to training sessions, hitting daily macronutrient requirements, and getting adequate sleep.

You also need to set goals that evaluate how near your behavior goals are taking you to your outcome goal. An example are strength goals. In the previous chapter, you learned that strength is important for building muscle and were given benchmarks to strive for. Reaching these strength benchmarks will show you how your muscle-building endeavors are going and make it easier for you to build and maintain muscle.

Since muscle is built in the gym, going to the gym is an important behavior goal. You need to determine how many times a week you can commit. Don't throw out a random number of days that your schedule can't possibly accommodate, as this sets you up to fail. Seriously check your Sunday-through-Saturday schedule for daily free blocks of from one to one and a half hours. Three such daily blocks a week is the minimum, but better results come with four days a week.

If you can, rearrange your schedule. Give up unimportant things. People claim, "I don't have time to workout," but then watch hours of TV. Make time to get to the gym and treat that time as if it's a doctor or dentist appointment. Make your behavior goals habits, and you'll easily reach your outcome goals.

Chapter 9:
How to Eat an Elephant

Strength coach Dan John famously teaches people seeking to build muscle how to eat an elephant. If the only way to free yourself and your family from kidnappers is to eat an elephant, how would you do it? You'd start chomping away, of course, one bite at a time. It would take you months, maybe years, but eventually you'd devour that elephant and be free.

Building muscle is a similarly long, slow progress. You realize as you look in the mirror that you've got a long way to go before achieving your dream physique. I assure you that you'll get there if you eat that elephant one bite at a time. Workout by workout, set by set, repetition by repetition, you will get there. Instead of contemplating how much you have yet to do when you look in the mirror, say to yourself, "Look at all the progress I've made since I started." The change in mindset that occurs will do wonders for your success.

For the best results, focus on getting stronger. Strength is the underlying theme of this book and is important in more ways than one. Your aim for every workout should be to equal or exceed your previous workout.

Each workout is a competition. Let's say your previous workout involved bench pressing as follows:

- Set 1: 135 lb. (61 kg) for 12 reps
- Set 2: 135 lb. for 11 reps
- Set 3: 135 lb. for 9 reps

That's 135 lb. lifted 32 total repetitions. At your next workout, you should bench press one of

1. 135 lb. for 32 total reps,
2. 135 lb. for 33 total reps, or
3. 140 lb. for 32 total reps.

No. 1 ties your previous performance, and Nos. 2 and 3 beat it by either increased repetitions or weight. This ensures constant strength gains and muscle building. I recommend doing No. 2 each workout until you are able to hoist 135 lb. for 36 total reps (3 sets of 12 reps).

Beating or tying your previous marker is known as the overload principle. At each session, you overload your muscles so they get bigger and stronger. It's eating the elephant one bite at a time. You might not want to train some days, but forcing yourself to do so and equaling or exceeding your previous performance is the only way to progress.

Chapter 10:
The FVI Most Wanted

Building muscle is similar to preparing great food. Each calls for a few key ingredients that make all the difference for a quality outcome. In building muscle, those ingredients are frequency, volume, and intensity (FVI). They work in together and separately.

Frequency is how often you train a muscle, volume is the total number of reps you work a muscle, and intensity is the extent to which you load a muscle. Manipulating these ingredients, individually and in combination, drastically changes your strength and muscle mass outcomes.

Frequency

This book gives you programs for training a body part once, twice, even three times a week. My theory is that training frequency relates to muscle protein synthesis (MPS), the building of proteins in your muscle. The more frequently you train, the more you boost MPS beyond the rate of muscle protein breakdown and, thus, the greater your muscle growth.

MPS is stimulated by resistance exercise and protein consumption; squats and steaks, if you will. Lifting weights elevates your MPS for 24–48 hours. So training 3–7 days per week will keep MPS high. Does this mean you can't train a body part once or twice per week? No, you can train a body part frequently and make fantastic gains. In fact, frequent training might be optimal.

Volume

Research shows that volume—10 sets of 10 reps of bench press is a volume of 100 reps—is one of the biggest drivers of muscle and strength. I think, however, that this needs qualification in light especially of the interrelationship between volume, frequency, and intensity. Doing 10 sets of 10 reps with 50 lb. (23 kg) and 10 sets of 10 reps with 100 lb. (45 kg) is equal in volume, at 100 reps, but a load of 100 lb. will elicit greater strength and muscle gains.

Intensity

The higher the load the greater the intensity, and the greater the intensity the higher the tension in the muscle. Tension, as we've seen, is one of three mechanisms for muscle growth. It is essential, therefore, to always consider intensity together with volume. We need to measure both the weight lifted and the total number of reps by multiplying the volume by the intensity (VI), as in the following examples:

$$VI = 10 \text{ sets} \times 10 \text{ reps} \times 50 \text{ lb. } (23 \text{ kg}) = 5,000 \text{ lb. } (2,268 \text{ kg})^*\text{reps}$$

$$VI = 10 \text{ sets} \times 10 \text{ reps} \times 100 \text{ lb. } (45 \text{ kg}) = 10,000 \text{ lb. } (4,536 \text{ kg})^*\text{reps}$$

I like this VI measurement because it allows you to quantify the tension going into the muscle and not just the total number of reps performed by the muscle. You want to do the minimum VI needed to reach your goal because one day you will plateau. If you can add 10 lb. (5 kg) of muscle to your legs in 10 weeks by squatting 200 lb. (91 kg) for 5 sets of 10 reps, there's no point doing more than 5 sets. Only when you plateau, will you need to raise your VI.

Frequency vs. Volume and Intensity

I recommend analyzing your VI weekly not daily to take into account frequency. Say you spread 10 sets of 10 reps over three workouts in a week instead of doing everything in a day. On Monday, you do 4 sets of 10 reps and then finish the week with 3 sets of 10 reps on each of Wednesday and Friday. Your total for the week remains 10 sets of 10 reps. And the heightened frequency keeps your MPS elevated throughout the week.

Another bonus to incorporating frequency into the VI equation is that you can employ higher intensities in each workout because you won't fatigue as much as you would doing 10 sets of 10 reps in a single workout. Increased weekly frequency, therefore, raises your VI. This translates into greater tension in and only moderate damage to muscle.

Training more frequently is great, but there is a con, and it's why many bodybuilders train a body part only once per week. Higher frequency sacrifices metabolic stress—the pump, or hypertrophy, in the muscle. If in a single workout you do 10 sets of 10 reps, your metabolic stress will be high, as will your muscle damage. Mechanical tension, though, will be low to moderate, and MPS will only be elevated once a week.

So which is better, training more frequently with a higher VI or training less frequently with a moderate VI but for greater metabolic stress and muscle damage? I prefer that drug-free lifters train frequently. Frequent training facilitates strength, and strength is what you need to build muscle.

Strength, moreover, is vital when you opt to build muscle using a low-frequency, high-daily volume routine. This, too, is an effective way of building muscle, which I also still advocate using. Low-frequency training does work, but it works best if you've acquired the strength that high-frequency training affords.

Reference

Damas, Felipe, et al. "A Review of Resistance Training-Induced Changes in Skeletal Muscle Protein Synthesis and Their Contribution to Hypertrophy." *Sports Medicine*, vol. 45, no. 6, 2015, pp. 801–807., doi:10.1007/s40279-015-0320-0.

Chapter 11:
How to Succeed

Ask the top bodybuilders of all time what the best program is for building muscle, and you'll get a different answer from each person. There are, as you'll see, many ways to gain muscle. The key, however, is that you must physically do the work regardless of the approach chosen.

Every bodybuilder thinks that his or her program is best. What many don't realize is that it's their adherence to the program and not the program itself that brings them success. You must comply with your program to ensure progress in the way of ongoing gains in muscle.

This chapter shows you how best to enhance your program adherence and progress.

Determine Your Personal Schedule

When you start training, you need to scrutinize your schedule. When do you work? When do you sleep? When do you have fun? When do you waste time? You must be honest and realistic, all the while looking for or arranging blocks of time for your important activities, including when you can go to the gym, grocery shop, rest and recover, and more. The aim is to make time for training and nutrition and all things required for building muscle and living well.

You may need to sacrifice one activity for another. The time you spend on the couch surfing social media sites or watching television might be better spent on more beneficial things. In the week ahead, record how you spend your time hourly. You'll see how much time you waste in a day and how you might find time to train on your lunch break or before or after work and possibly over the weekend.

How to Make Time

Among the strategies you can use to clear your schedule, I recommend batching your time for a particular activity and avoiding multitasking, where you waste time switching between tasks. Focus on and finish one task before moving to another.

- Do your laundry 1–2 times a week instead of on numerous, nearly daily occasions.
- Check your e-mail once a day instead of frequently throughout the day.
- Wash all of your dishes once a day instead of after each meal prep or meal.
- Shop for groceries once a week instead of every day.

- Prepare a large amount of food 1–2 times a week for lunches instead of daily.

Another method to make time is to buy it. Pay others to do tasks around your home, including cleaning, gardening, cooking, and so on. Provided you earn more per hour than the person you hire, this a terrific way to free up time throughout the week. And that's worth the cost.

Track Progress

Once you start your training program, track your progress. Weigh yourself; measure your body parts; record the loads, sets, and reps for each lift you perform.

I recommend tracking your body weight weekly. This number gives you solid data on your muscle-building progress. When I started my fitness journey, I was 155 lb (70 kg). As of writing this, I'm fluctuating between 185 (84 kg) and 190 lb. (86 kg). I wish I'd tracked my weight to see all the changes over the past nine years.

The best time of day to weigh yourself is in the morning upon waking, after using the bathroom and before drinking or eating. Consistency in this respect ensures accurate data.

Measure the circumference of the following body parts at the start of each month:

- Arms
- Calves
- Neck
- Thighs
- Waist
- Chest
- Shoulders
- Forearms

At the gym, write down in a notebook every set and rep and load for each lift you execute. This way, you'll see your progress unfold, page by page.

You'll find that tracking your progress is good motivation. This process is key in focusing you on how far you've come instead of on how far you have to go. Training needs to be a positive thing, and emphasizing good instead of bad news will make you happy and further your adherence to the program.

Support Network

Author and motivational speaker Jim Rohn said that "you are the average of the five people you spend the most time with." In other words, if your friends and family are obese, you'll probably be obese too. I knew a girl, in fact, who exercised and was lean but who started hanging out with a group of obese friends after moving to a new city. A few months of weekend pizzas and cola, and she unsurprisingly gained 20 lb. (9 kg). Alternatively, a slightly overweight friend of mine moved in with me during university, started working out and eating better, and lost 10–15 lb. (5–7 kg). It works both ways.

To help you reach your goals, you need to cultivate a support network. Find a gym buddy and hold each other accountable. Go to the gym with your significant other and eat healthy food together. Cut off unhealthy friendships in exchange for healthy ones.

Progressive Overload

Follow the progressive overload principle, as it ensures that you get stronger each workout. Keep in mind that you're not training to build muscle but, rather, to develop the strength to build muscle. It doesn't matter if you're using high reps or low reps. Your goal is to increase the amount of weight your lift. Your goal for every workout is to beat or tie what you did in your previous workout. If in one workout you bench press 100 lb. (45 kg) for 30 total reps, your aim in the next workout involving bench press is one of the following:

- 100 lb. (45 kg) for 30 total reps (ties previous workout)
- 100 lb. (45 kg) for 31 total reps (beats previous workout)
- 105 lb. (48 kg) for 30 total reps (beats previous workout)

Do not sacrifice form for weight. This is why you will sometimes have to tie your previous performance. The key is to make progress bit by bit, workout by workout, week by week. This ensures that you are overloading your muscles. It tells them they need to grow stronger.

SECTION 2:
PUMPING IRON

Chapter 12:
How to Train

This is the section of the book you've been waiting for: the muscle-building program. I need first, however, to teach you how to succeed on the program. This includes instructions on how to read the workouts, when to train, and how much weight to use.

How to Read the Workouts

Workouts utilize terms that you need to understand to ensure correct performance of the program. It's a written language that translates into you moving your body and building muscle.

Rep is short for repetition and refers to a single performance of a single exercise.

Set is the total number of repetitions performed without stopping.

Tempo refers to the speed at which one repetition is performed. It's denoted by four numbers, such as 4-0-1-0. Each number represents the seconds to complete a phase of the movement. The first number represents the eccentric phase (lowering the weight to the ground), the second is the pause, the third is the concentric phase (moving the weight from the ground), and the fourth is the pause.

For the bench press, for example, the first number cited above, 4, indicates 4 seconds to lower the weight eccentrically to the chest. The second number, 0, is how long to pause the bar at the chest. The third, 1, is the speed in seconds for concentrically pressing the bar upward. The fourth, 0, is the length of the pause at the top of the press.

Occasionally, an X will appear for a lift's concentric phase in the four-number series. The X instructs you to explode on the concentric phase of a lift. If the weight is heavy, your explosion may take several seconds. Just push as hard as you can, maintaining tension in the muscle being worked—the pecs in the case of the bench press.

Rest is the time between sets.

1A and 1B, etc., refer to the order of exercises. 1A is the first exercise for a particular set for a particular body part, while 1B refers to the second exercise. After completing 1A, rest for the amount of time predetermined in the program and then do exercise 1B. Rest again for the predetermined time and then perform the second set of exercise 1A.

Putting It All Together

Following is a sample workout to teach you how to read the terminology above within a typical workout format. Do not do this workout; it is intended as an example only.

Exercise	Sets	Reps	Rest (sec)	Tempo
1A: Bench Press	2	5	60	40X0
1B: Pull-ups	2	5	120	4011
2: Squats	3	6	180	3310
3A: Over-head Press	2	8	60	2010
3B: Biceps Curl	2	8	45	2010
3C: Triceps Press down	2	8	30	2010

1A and 1B: Bench Press and Pull-ups

Start with 5 repetitions of bench press. Each rep involves 4 seconds of lowering the bar, no pause, an explosive pushing of the bar upward, and no pause. Five continuous reps equal one set. Rest 60 seconds and move to exercise 1B: pull-ups.

Do 5 reps of pull-ups. Each rep involves 4 seconds of lowering yourself, no pause, 1 second of pulling yourself up to the bar, and 1 second of holding yourself at the top of the movement. Five continuous reps equal one set. Rest 120 seconds, then do a second set of bench press followed by a second set of pull-ups before moving to exercise 2: squats.

2: Squats

Do squats for 6 repetitions. One repetition involves 3 seconds of lowering yourself, 3 seconds of holding the bottom position, 1 second of rising to the start position, and no pause. Six continuous reps is one set. Rest 180 seconds and repeat for a total of 3 sets. Then move to exercise 3A: overhead press.

3A, 3B, and 3C: Overhead Press, Biceps Curls, and Triceps Push down

Do 8 repetitions of overhead press. One repetition involves 1 second of pressing the weight overhead followed without pause by 2 seconds of lowering the weight and no pause. Eight continuous reps is one set. Rest 60 seconds and switch to exercise 3B: biceps curls.

Do 8 repetitions of biceps curls. Each repetition involves 1 second to curl the weight up, no pause, 2 seconds to lower the weight, and no pause. Eight continuous reps is one set. Rest 45 seconds, then go to exercise 3C: triceps push down.

Do 8 repetitions of triceps press down. Each repetition involves pressing the handle down for 1 second followed immediately by 2 seconds of letting the handle come back up and no pause. Eight continuous reps is one set. Rest 30 seconds, then do a second set of the overhead press (3A) followed by a second set of each of exercises 3B and 3C.

As you can see, there is a small learning curve to reading a workout. But you'll soon be able to follow any program.

When to Train

In the workouts to come, you'll notice that each has a different number of training days, ranging from two days to six days per week. You'll also notice that I offer workout schedules. These are suggested schedules only; the proposed days will not fit everyone's calendars. If a four-day program tells you to work out on Sunday, Monday, Wednesday, and Friday, by all means chose other days if one or more of my suggested days doesn't suit. But do stick with the four-day-a-week regimen or with whatever regimen is prescribed for a specific workout.

How Much Weight to Use

Should you use heavy weights or light weights? The answer is simple: go as heavy as you can without breaking form or dropping reps. Different exercises call for different rep ranges. You need to lift as much weight as you can while ensuring that you complete the predetermined number of repetitions with good form. If you can't do all the reps because of fatigue and form breakdown, the weight is too heavy.

Let's say a workout calls for 5 reps of bench press. You need to find a weight at which you can do the 5 reps without loss of form. If you bench press 210 lb. (95 kg) and can do only 4 reps with perfect form, you're lifting too much weight. Conversely, if you use 190 lb. (86 kg) and feel that you could do more than 5 reps, the weight is too light. Bench pressing 200 lb. (91 kg) for 5 reps with solid form means you're using an appropriate weight.

But what about if you need to bench press 15 reps? That 200 lb. will be inappropriate. You'll again need to find a weight that allows you to execute a good 15 reps.

Progressing, of course, means that you'll need to eventually lift more weight or do more reps. Here's what I recommend. Each workout, try to beat or tie the weight you used for a lift previously. Say you were able to bench press 200 lb. for 3 sets of 5 reps last workout. At your next workout, try to do either 3 sets of 6 reps at 200 lb. or 1 set of 5 reps at 205 lb. (92 kg). If you select the greater weight option and can only bench press 3–4 reps in sets 2 and 3, this is fine. I will explain more about this later.

Chapter 13:
Warming Up

What do most people do before a workout? They jump on the treadmill for 5–10 minutes to warm up. After reading this chapter, you will never warm up on a treadmill again.

I believe that a proper warm-up can help you build muscle. A warm-up should both elevate your body temperature and enhance your mobility. That combination decreases your risk of injury, in and out of the gym. If you can't train because of injury, you're not going to be able to build muscle. Think of the warm-up as your injury insurance.

The warm-up you are about to learn has three phases: mobility, activation, and breathing. These should be done before every workout. The warm-up also includes exercise warm-up sets that are to be done before the first several exercises of every workout.

Mobility

Building muscle requires you to lift a weight through a full range of motion. If your mobility is compromised, this will be difficult. Some body parts, such as the ankles, hips, and upper back and shoulders, have large ranges of motion. Others don't, including your knees, lower back, and elbows. The mobility phase aims in particular to increase and maintain the mobility of your ankles, hips, and upper back and shoulders.

Quadruped Rocking (Hips)

1. Start on your hands and knees. Your hands should be shoulder width apart, and your knees should be slightly wider than shoulder width apart.
2. Turn your butt up (like a stripper showing off her butt).
3. Brace your core (as if getting ready to be punched in the stomach).
4. Rock your hips backward toward your heels while bracing your core and maintaining your upturned butt.
5. Repeat 10–12 times.

Quadruped Extension Rotation (Upper back and shoulders)

1. Start on your hands and knees. Your hands and knees should be shoulder width apart.
2. Cup your right hand behind your head.
3. Brace your core (as if getting ready to be punched in the stomach).
4. Bring your right elbow down toward your left hand (within 15–20 cm).

5. Then move your right elbow up toward the ceiling.

6. Repeat 10–12 times for the right side and then the left side.

Downward Dog (Ankles)

1. Start on your hands and knees. Your hands and knees should be shoulder width apart.

2. Feet on the floor, lift your knees off the floor.

3. Straighten your legs and upper body and push your butt up as high as possible (forming a triangle with the floor).

4. Press your heels to the floor (you should feel a stretch in the hamstrings and calves).

5. Hold this position for 30 seconds.

Activation

The best way to lock in your mobility gains is through activation. Activation trains your body for a strong range of motion by doing more than simply stretching the muscle and then allowing it to return to its previous, static state.

Single-Leg Deadlift to Reverse Lunge

1. Stand up straight with both feet together.

2. Raise your right leg backward while reaching forward with your right hand. Keep the right leg and arm extended to form a straight line

parallel with the floor (your body will make a
T with your legs).

3. Hold this position for 5 seconds and then stand
up straight again.

4. Step backward with your right leg into a deep
lunge.

5. Hold this position for 5 seconds.

6. Use your right leg to stand up straight.

7. Repeat for 3 repetitions on the right side and
then the left side.

Deep Iso Squat

1. Stand up straight with your feet shoulder
width apart.

2. Hold your hands together as if you are about
to pray.

3. Push apart your knees and squat down
between your knees until the pointy part of
your elbow touches the meaty party of your
inner thigh.

4. Stay in this deep squat and push your knees
apart with your elbows.

5. Hold this position for 30 seconds.

Prone V Raise

1. Lie face down onto the floor.

2. Extend your arms over your head to form the
Y in YMCA.

3. Point your thumbs to the ceiling and lift your hands 5 cm off the floor.
4. Hold that position for 2 seconds.
5. Lower your arms to the floor.
6. Repeat for 10 repetitions.

Breathing

Breathing properly is the most important thing you can learn. Many of the aches and pains that we experience can be fixed simply by retraining ourselves to breathe correctly for the 17,000 to 30,000 breaths we take per day.

How do you breathe properly? Breathe with your diaphragm. For exemplary breathing, watch babies. Their abdomens puff out as they inhale. Adults often suck in their abdomens to make themselves appear lean. This causes them to breathe only with their upper chest and trapezius muscles. The result is shoulder, neck, and back tension and pain, including headaches.

Practice breathing before every workout using the following routine:

Supine Diaphragmatic Breathing

1. Lie on your back.
2. Place one hand on your abdomen (below the belly button) and one hand on your chest.
3. Inhale deeply by pushing your abdomen to the ceiling.
4. Exhale by drawing your abdomen back in.
5. The hand on your abdomen should move up and down. The hand on your chest should not.
6. Do this for 10–20 breaths.

Warm-up Sets

Unlike the mobility, activation, and breathing phases, which are done before workouts, the warm-up sets are exercise specific and meant to be done prior to actual workout exercises. They are practice movements of workout exercises employing light loads to set you up to perform those exercises with heavy loads.

I recommend doing a warm-up set for the first two or three exercises of a workout. This gets blood into the muscle and increases your body temperature locally for a lift. Say, for example, your first exercise is bench press for 10 reps. You know that you can bench press 185 lb. (84 kg) for 10 reps, but to warm-up you're not going to throw 185 lb. on the bar and lift for 10 reps. You're going to work your way up to that weight through three warm-up sets as follows:

- Bench press the bar for 10 reps.
- Rest 1 min.
- Bench press 95 lb. (43 kg) for 10 reps.
- Rest 2 min.
- Bench press 155 lb. (70 kg) for 8 reps.
- Rest 2–3 min.
- Proceed to fully loaded exercise.

You can see above that your first warm-up set involves lifting only an unloaded bar. If your first exercise involves dumbbells, use lightly loaded dumbbells. Again, the purpose of these warm-up sets is merely to prepare for the movement.

The second set should involve the full number of reps but at a load close to 50% of what your actual lift load. The third and last warm-up set should involve a weight that is about 80% of your actual lift weight and 2 reps less than the full number of predetermined reps. In our example above, the third warm-up set is 8 reps in place of the 10 prescribed. If a workout calls for 5 reps, your third warm-up set will be 3 reps, and so on. Using this method prepares your body for the work to come.

Chapter 14:
Your Muscle-Building Recipe

The *Muscle* program offers you a choose-your-own-workouts approach. Everyone is different, so everyone needs a different plan of action to get where they want to get. There are, however, a few rules to follow for the perfect plan.

Chief among them is that you are always training for strength. It doesn't matter if your outcome goal is to build muscle, lose fat, specialize, base build, or maintain. You need to think of the gym as a place to get strong. Your aim is always to do one more repetition or to increase the load. To gain strength, you need tension in the muscle. This will tell your muscle to grow. Provided you adhere to this book's workouts and work daily to get strong, you will build muscle.

In subsequent chapters, you'll find the following training phases:

- **Base Building** will build a strong and well-balanced body. You will do a lot of different things to help prep you for the workouts. This includes core work, full-body training, and injury prevention. Everyone should start with base building regardless of skill and should base build for 12 weeks a year.

- **Beginner Strength and Mass** gets you strong to build muscle and muscle mass with ease. You can't build muscle unless you're strong. Use this phase to add your first 20–30 lb. (9–14 kg) of it.

- **Intermediate Strength and Mass** builds on the previous phase to add another 20-30 lb. of muscle.

- **Advanced Strength and Mass** builds on the previous phase for ongoing muscle gains.

- **Specialization** hones in on those body parts that we all have that develop more slowly than others to bring it into proportion with the rest of your body.

- **Maintenance** preserves the dream body that you've built through the previous phases.

This book includes a few done-for-you programs for each phase. Choose one that works best for you and use it for the recommended period before moving on to another program or phase. Just be sure to include the key phases of base building, strength and mass, specialization, and maintenance in tailoring a training program for yourself.

To assist you, I will next provide overviews of sample plans for beginner, intermediate, and advanced trainees. These plans may be confusing because they reference programs for each of the training phases, and you may need to cross-reference from chapter to chapter to make sense of things. Read this and the chapters to come—on base building, strength and mass, specialization, and maintenance—and then reread this chapter for greater understand.

The Beginner Plan of Action

If you're just starting out and not very strong or have been lifting for fewer than two years and are yet to gain your first 20-30 lb. (9–14 kg) of muscle, I recommend the following approach:

Beginner Year 1

- Pick either a three- or four-day-a-week, done-for-you base-building program and do it for 12 weeks.
- Use a beginner strength and mass program for the rest of the year.

End of beginner year 1, muscle gained: 20–25 lb. (9–11 kg)

Beginner Year 2

- You need to base build once a year, so you'll be base building for the first 12 weeks of your second year of training.
- For the rest of the training year, use the intermediate strength and mass program.

End of beginner year 2, muscle gained: 10–12 lb. (4.5–5 kg); 30–37 lb. (14–16 kg) max

The Intermediate Plan of Action

If you've been lifting for more than two years; have satisfactory strength levels (see the "Intermediate Strength and Mass" chapter); and have gained 30 lb. (14 kg) of muscle, you are an intermediate. Your goal is to continue to build your strength from satisfactory to strong, as mentioned in the "How Strong Is Strong Enough?" chapter. I recommend this approach:

Intermediate Year 1

- Pick either a three- or four-day-a-week, done-for-you base-building program and do it for 12 weeks.
- For the rest of the training year, use the intermediate strength and mass program.

End of intermediate year 1, muscle gained: 5–6 lb. (2–3 kg)

Intermediate Year 2

- Same as previous year.

End of intermediate year 2, muscle gained: 2–3 lb. (1–1.4 kg)

The Advanced Plan of Action

If you've been lifting for more than four years, are strong as defined in the "How Strong Is Strong Enough? chapter, and have made great progress with your body, you can consider yourself advanced. Your goal is to raise yourself from strong to aesthetically strong and to specialize to bring lagging body parts into proportion. I recommend this approach:

Advanced Year 1

- Pick either a three- or four-day-a-week, done-for-you base-building program and do it for 12 weeks.
- For the rest of the training year, cycle between the advanced strength and mass and the specialization phases. Do each phase for 8–16 weeks before switching as follows:
  - Advanced strength and mass for 16 weeks
  - Specialization phase for 8 weeks
  - Advanced strength and mass for 16 weeks
  - Specialization phase for 8 weeks

Advanced Year 2 and Beyond

- You are now 8 weeks into the second year of your advanced plan. Continue using the previous year's approach until you are aesthetically strong. This could take 2–6 years.

The Maintenance Phase

Once you are happy with your body, you'll want to enter the maintenance phase. Happiness with your body means that you've reached your goal and wouldn't change anything. Some people reading this book may well be happy with the body they build after a single year of training. So be it. They then can enter the maintenance phase. Other people, conversely, set the bar extremely high and continue building their bodies for years to come before they enter the maintenance phase.

Everyone has different goals. Just ask yourself, am I happy with my body? If the answer is "yes," it's time to enter the maintenance phase.

Chapter 15:
Base Building

Building muscle, as with any endeavor, calls for establishing a base that sets you up for long-term success. You must build a base of key lifts that you rely on for strength gains and maintenance. You must also increase your movement capacity so that you can readily adapt to new lifts and athletic activities generally across a full range of motion, further your general conditioning and strength to enable you to handle higher volumes of work, develop sound techniques to prevent injury and the need for you to take time off training, and so on.

Base building should be done at the outset of every training year for a period of 12 weeks.

Base-Building Features
- Become expert in key lifts (compound unilateral and bilateral movements)
- Increase movement capacity
- Practice sound technique as injury prevention
- Improve general conditioning
- Do once a year as mandatory, 3–4 days per week for 12 weeks

The Base-Building Program

My program for base building is founded on things I learned in my first personal training job in Toronto. These fundamentals have stuck with me, and I find myself returning to them time and again because they are effective. The program can be done three days a week or four days a week using the following proposed schedules:

3–Day-per-Week Proposed Schedule

Sunday	Monday	Tuesday	Wednesday	Thursday	Friday	Saturday
	Workout A		Workout B		Workout A	
	Workout B		Workout A		Workout B	
	Workout A		Workout B		Workout A	
	Workout B		Workout A		Workout B	

4–Day-per-Week Proposed Schedule

Sunday	Monday	Tuesday	Wednesday	Thursday	Friday	Saturday
	Workout A	Workout B		Workout C		Workout D
	Workout A	Workout B		Workout C		Workout D

Weeks 1–4

Workout A

Exercise	Sets	Reps	Rest (sec)	Tempo
1: Front Plank	2	Hold for 60 seconds	60	n/a
2A: Goblet Squat	3	12	60	3010
2B: Quadruped Pull down	3	12 each arm	60	3010
3A: Dumbbell Step-up	3	12 each leg	60	3010
3B: Half-Kneel-ing Single-Arm Dumbbell Press	3	12 each arm	60	3010
Cardio Equip-ment of Choice	Go hard for 10 minutes straight.			

Workout B

Exercise	Sets	Reps	Rest (sec)	Tempo
1: Side Plank	2	Hold for 30 seconds on each side	60	n/a
2A: Cable Ro-manian Dead-lift	3	12	60	3010
2B: Push-up (add weight if necessary)	3	12 each arm	60	3010
3A: Split Squat	3	12 each leg	60	3010
3B: Quadruped Row	3	12 each arm	60	3010
Cardio Equip-ment of Choice	Do 5 rounds of intervals, doing each round as hard as you can for 60 seconds and then resting fully (do nothing) for 60 seconds before the next round.			

Weeks 5–8

Workout A

Exercise	Sets	Reps	Rest (sec)	Tempo
1: Forward Crawl	2	15–20 meters	60	n/a
2A: Front Squat	3-4	10	60	3010
2B: Lat Pull down or Chin-up	3-4	10	60	3010
3A: Single-Leg Cable Romanian Deadlift	3-4	10 each leg	60	3010
3B: Standing Dumbbell Press	3-4	10	60	3010
Cardio Equipment of Choice	Go hard for 10 minutes straight.			

Workout B

Exercise	Sets	Reps	Rest (sec)	Tempo
1: Single-Arm Farmer Carry	2	15–20 meters each arm	60	n/a
2A: Barbell Romanian Deadlift	3-4	10	60	3010
2B: Dumbbell Bench Press	3-4	10 each arm	60	3010
3A: Reverse Lunge	3-4	10 each leg	60	3010
3B: Single-Arm Cable Row	3-4	10 each arm	60	3010
Cardio Equipment of Choice	Do 10 rounds of intervals, doing each round as hard as you can for 30 seconds and then resting fully (do nothing) for 30 seconds before the next round.			

Cardio Equipment of Choice	Do 5 rounds of intervals, doing each round as hard as you can for 60 seconds and then resting fully (do nothing) for 60 seconds before the next round.

Weeks 9–12

Workout A

Exercise	Sets	Reps	Rest (sec)	Tempo
1: Backward Crawl	2	15–20 meters	60	n/a
2A: Back Squat	4	8	60	3010
2B: Lat Pull down or Chin-up	4	8	60	3010
3A: Single-Leg Dumbbell Romanian Deadlift	4	8 each leg	60	3010
3B: Barbell Military Press	4	8	60	3010
Cardio Equipment of Choice	Go hard for 10 minutes straight.			

Workout B

Exercise	Sets	Reps	Rest (sec)	Tempo
1: Heavy Farmer Carry	2	15–20 meters	60	n/a
2A: Rack Pull from Knees	4	8	60	3010
2B: Barbell Bench Press	4	8	60	3010
3A: Bulgarian Split Squat	4	8 each leg	60	3010
3B: Chest Supported Row	4	8	60	3010
Bike Intervals	Do 5 rounds of intervals, doing each round as hard as you can for 15 seconds against a decent resistance and then resting fully (do nothing) for 105 seconds before the next round.			

A Note on Cardio

The goal with cardio is to condition your heart to be strong (there's that word again). This will benefit you in two ways:

1. A strong heart will help you in day-to-day activities, such as cutting the lawn, shoveling snow, moving furniture, or walking up a long flight of stairs.
2. A strong heart will increase your work capacity when you lift weights. Ever gotten tired after doing high-rep sets? Having a strong heart will make sure that your muscles fail before your heart does.

In almost all instances, I say "use cardio equipment of choice." This means you can use any cardio equipment or method you can think of and that appeals to you. Here are a few options:

- Exercise bike
- Treadmill
- Step Climber
- Rowing Machine
- Push Sled
- Sprinting/Running
- Battle Ropes
- Burpees

For workout B of weeks 9–12, I specify "bike intervals." I do this because there is new research showing that Wingate sprints done on a stationary bike are extremely beneficial for fat loss and for conditioning your heart to recover. For maximum benefit, however, you must do the bike intervals as hard as you possibly can for 15 seconds. And you'll want to do them using a decent resistance on the bike. The goal is for your legs to be going fast against resistance for 15 seconds. If you do this correctly, you may feel a bit nauseous.

What about Arms and Calves?

You may notice that base building doesn't have any direct arm or calf work. This is because the goal is to get you stronger in a few key lifts for total body effectiveness. You can, though, do the following at the end of your workouts:

Day A Arms Option

Exercise	Sets	Reps	Rest (sec)	Tempo
1: Biceps Exercise of Choice	3–4	8–12	60	3010
2: Triceps Exercise of Choice	3–4	8–12	60	3010

Day B Calves Option

Exercise	Sets	Reps	Rest (sec)	Tempo
1: Standing Calf Raises	3–4	10–15	60	3010
2: Seated Calf Raises	3–4	15–20	60	3010

Chapter 16:
Beginner Strength and Mass

Next to base building, strength workouts are the most important. If you're strong, lifting weights burns calories, and you'll find it easier to stay lean, which is important because you want your waist to be small. If you're strong, moreover, you can lift heavy weights to aid in your focus on hypertrophy (muscle building), enabling you to build muscle faster and keep it longer.

The workouts in this phase are not only for strength. They also build muscle mass; this book is called *Muscle* after all. There's no point striving solely to increase your one repetition maximum. You'll want to build muscle in the process. Remember, mechanical tension builds muscle. These workouts oblige by providing a lot of tension. So in a nutshell, this phase builds strength first and muscle mass second.

The strength and mass phase should only be done after you've completed the base-building phase. And you should continue doing the strength aspect of the phase until your strength levels are satisfactory. For some people this could take a couple months. Others may require a year. It all depends on how strong you are at the start and on how quickly your body responds.

If you'll recall, I provided strength goals in the "How Strong Is Strong Enough?" chapter. These are the goals you'll be working toward in this phase. Do not move on to the mass, or hypertrophy, aspect of the phase (next chapter) until you have satisfactory strength, the goals for which are 80% of the strong category. For your convenience, I've included the satisfactory strength targets below.

Exercise	Strength Goal (1RM)
Bench Press	1 x body weight
Single-Arm Bench Press	0.4 x body weight
Weighted Chin-up	0.48 x body weight
Barbell Military Press	0.64 x body weight
Single-Arm Dumbbell Military Press	0.267 x body weight
Back Squat	1.32 x body weight
Bulgarian Split Squat	0.8 x body weight
Deadlift	1.6 x body weight
Single-Leg Deadlift	1.08 x body weight

To summarize, continue using the workouts in this chapter until you have reached the satisfactory strength goals above. You need to be satisfactory in either a bilateral or unilateral exercise, but both is best. Make sure to follow "The Plan" chapter to see your entire *Muscle* journey.

Beginner Strength and Mass Key Features

- Get strong first
- Build dense muscle
- Do 3–4 days per week
- Lengthen rest periods the heavier the weight
- Use to reach satisfactory strength levels
- Gain first 20–30 lb. (9–14 kg) of muscle

Workout Flow

The workouts are meant to be simple. You'll start each training session by strengthening your core muscles. This will train your abs and prime your core for the heavy lifting ahead.

After core work, you get into the meat and potatoes of the workout: strength work. You will train your full body with superset exercises to maximize your time in the gym. Remember to use progressive overload to ensure strength gains.

There are two exercises for each of the compound movements of horizontal push, horizontal pull, vertical push, vertical pull, knee dominant, and hip dominant. One exercise is bilateral to train both sides together and the other exercise is unilateral to train each side separately. This will ensure that you build a balanced body.

You then have the option to isolate body parts and muscles, such as arms, rear delts, and calves. If you don't like doing isolation work, skip it.

Beginner Muscle Schedule

You have two workout schedule options: three days a week or every other day. Use the schedule that works best for you. Just make sure you take at least one day off following a day of training.

Option 1: 3 Days per Week

Sun-day	Monday	Tues-day	Wednes-day	Thurs-day	Friday	Satur-day
	Workout A		Workout B		Workout A	
	Workout B		Workout A		Workout B	
	Workout A		Workout B		Workout A	
	Workout B		Workout A		Workout B	

Option 2: Every Other Day

Sunday	Mon-day	Tues-day	Wednes-day	Thurs-day	Friday	Satur-day
Workout A		Workout B		Workout A		Workout B
	Workout A		Workout B		Workout A	
Workout B		Workout A		Workout B		Workout A
	Workout B		Workout A		Workout B	

Beginner Muscle Workout A

Core

Exercise	Sets	Reps	Rest (seconds)
Front Plank	2	Hold for 60 seconds	60

Strength

Exercise	Sets	Reps	Rest (seconds)
1A: Front Squat	3	8–10	60
1B: Chin-up or Lat Pull down	3	8–10	60
2A: Single-Leg Romanian Deadlift	3	8–10 each leg	60
2B: Dumbbell Military Press	3	8–10	60
3A: Barbell Bench Press	3	8–10	60
3B: Single-Arm Dumbbell Row	3	8–10 each arm	60

Isolation (Optional)

Exercise	Sets	Reps	Rest (seconds)
1: Calf Raises	3	8–10	60
2: Rear Delt Flys	3	8–10	60

Beginner Muscle Workout B

Core

Exercise	Sets	Reps	Rest (seconds)
Side Plank	2	Hold for 30 seconds on each side	60

Strength

Exercise	Sets	Reps	Rest (seconds)
1A: Rack Deadlift	3	8–10	60
1B: Dumbbell Bench Press	3	8–10	60
2A: Bulgarian Split Squat	3	8–10 each leg	60
2B: Chest-Supported Dumbbell Row	3	8–10	60
3A: Barbell Military Press	3	8–10	60
3B: Single-Arm Lat Pull down	3	8–10 each arm	60

Isolation (Optional)

Exercise	Sets	Reps	Rest (seconds)
1: Dumbbell Biceps Curls	3	8–10	60
2: Cable Triceps Press down	3	8–10	60

Milk Your Newbie Gains

As a beginner, you're going to experience some amazing newbie gains. You'll basically get stronger every workout and pack on muscle easily if you embrace the overload principle.

Milk your newbie gains for as long as you can with full-body workouts until they stop working. Your goal is to build muscle, so don't stop doing whatever achieves that goal.

I recommend doing a full-body routine until you've gained your first 20 lb. (9 kg) of muscle. But if you're still gaining, keep going with full-body work.

When either you've gained your first 20 lb. of muscle or the full-body program stops working, it's time for you to graduate to intermediate-level workouts.

Chapter 17:
Intermediate Strength and Mass

If you've been lifting for more than two years, have satisfactory strength, and have gained 30 lb. (14 kg) of muscle, you are an intermediate. Your goal is to achieve the strong category mentioned in the "How Strong Is Strong Enough?" chapter.

Exercise	Strength Goal (1RM)
Bench Press	1.25 x body weight
Single-Arm Bench Press	0.5 x body weight
Weighted Chin-up	0.6 x body weight
Barbell Military Press	0.8 x body weight
Single-Arm Dumbbell Military Press	0.333 x body weight
Back Squat	1.65 x body weight
Bulgarian Split Squat	1 x body weight
Deadlift	2 x body weight
Single-Leg Deadlift	1.35 x body weight

To summarize, continue with the intermediate strength and mass phase until you reach the strong goals in the table above. Make sure to review "The Plan" chapter for an overview of your *Muscle* journey.

Intermediate Strength and Mass Key Features

- Get strong first
- Build dense muscle
- Do 3–4 days per week
- Lengthen rest periods the heavier the weight

- Use to reach strong levels
- Gain next 10–17 lb. (5–8 kg) of muscle.

Inspired by "The Shadow"

In the 1990s, pro bodybuilder Dorian Yates, "the Shadow," was known as one of the biggest and leanest bodybuilders ever. His quiet yet intense persona arose from his documentary *Blood & Guts*, in which he trained to all-out failure, screaming up a lung in black-and-white glory.

Yates was famous for his blood and guts one set to all-out failure approach. It was copied by many beginner and intermediate trainees, who were disappointed with the results. It just didn't work. The truth is, even Dorian Yates didn't use the one set to all-out failure approach until he was already a world champion bodybuilder. He built his body on an upper-lower split. In fact, Yates used a full-body routine until he weighed 180 lb. (82 kg) and then switched to an upper-lower split to get to 220 lb. (100 kg). And most of his gains were natural, involving no steroids.

The intermediate plan to follow is based on what Yates did to go from 180 lb. to 220 lb. Yates's four-set approach of two warm-up sets and two work sets are ideal for intermediate trainees.

Here's how what we'll call the 4-set method is going to work in the intermediate plan:

- Set 1 (Warm-up): 50% of your work set
- Set 2 (Warm-up): 70–75% of your work set
- Set 3 (Work Set): 100% of your work set
- Set 4 (Back-off Set): 90% of your work set

If you plan to bench press 200 lb. (91 kg) for 8 reps, your four sets will look like this:

- Set 1 (Warm-up): 50% of your work set, or 100 lb. (45 kg) for 8 reps
- Set 2 (Warm-up): 70–75% of your work set, or 140–150 lb. (64–68 kg) for 8 reps
- Set 3 (Work Set): 100% of your work set, or 200 lb. (91 kg) for 8 reps
- Set 4 (Back-off Set): 90% of your work set, or 180 lb. (82 kg) for 8 reps

The overload principle is built into every workout, so you are always building. Remember, work set 3 is key. The 4-set method, moreover, has a strength day and a hypertrophy day.

On strength days, you'll lift in the 4–6 rep range. Let's say you can deadlift 300 lb. (136 kg) for 5 reps. Apply the 4-set method to deadlifting that weight for that number of reps in a workout. The next time you deadlift, your goal will be 6 reps using the 4-set method. Once you can do 6 reps, your next deadlift workout should see you add 5 lb. (2 kg) and start at 4 reps. Here's the set 3 progression for strength-day workouts:

Exercise	Week 1	Week 2	Week 3	Week 4	Week 5	Week 6
Deadlift	300 lb. (136 kg) for 5 reps	300 lb. for 6 reps	305 lb. (138 kg) for 4 reps	305 lb. for 5 reps	305 lb. for 6 reps	310 lb. (141 kg) for 4 reps

This progression, as you can see, has overload built in. On set 3 of week 1, you'll aim for 300 lb. for 5 reps, on set 3 of week 2, you'll aim for 300 lb. for 6 reps, and so on.

On hypertrophy days, you'll lift in the 6–8 rep range under the 4-set method. Using the dumbbell military press as an example, a hypertrophy day might look like this:

Exercise	Week 1	Week 2	Week 3	Week 4	Week 5	Week 6
Dumbbell Military Press	55 lb. (25 kg) for 6 reps	55 lb. for 7 reps	55 lb. for 8 reps	60 lb. (27 kg) for 6 reps	60 lb. for 7 reps	60 lb. for 8 reps

Again, keep in mind that the weights used above are for set 3 of the 4-set method. Here's how week 1 would look:

- Set 1 (Warm-up): 50% of your work set, or 30 lb. (14 kg) for 6 reps
- Set 2 (Warm-up): 70–75% of your work set, or 40 lb. (18 kg) for 6 reps
- Set 3 (Work Set): 100% of your work set, or 55 lb. (25 kg) for 6 reps
- Set 4 (Back-off Set): 90% of your work set, or 50 lb. (23 kg) for 6 reps

Week 6 would look as follows:

- Set 1 (Warm-up): 50% of your work set, or 30 lb. (14 kg) for 8 reps
- Set 2 (Warm-up): 70–75% of your work set, or 45 lb. (20 kg) for 8 reps
- Set 3 (Work Set): 100% of your work set, or 60 lb. (27 kg) for 8 reps
- Set 4 (Back-off Set): 90% of your work set, or 55 lb. (25 kg) for 8 reps

Intermediate Strength and Mass Schedule

You have two workout schedule options for developing intermediate strength and mass: 3 days a week or 4 days a week. If your recovery is poor, work out three days a week, but I'd try both schedules. Settle on the schedule that works best for you.

Option 1: 3 Days per Week

Sunday	Monday	Tuesday	Wednesday	Thursday	Friday	Saturday
	Upper Strength		Lower Strength		Upper Hypertrophy	
	Lower Hypertrophy		Upper Strength		Lower Strength	
	Upper Hypertrophy		Lower Hypertrophy		Upper Strength	
	Lower Strength		Upper Hypertrophy		Lower Hypertrophy	

Option 2: 4 Days per Week

Sunday	Monday	Tuesday	Wednesday	Thursday	Friday	Saturday
Upper Strength	Lower Strength		Upper Hypertrophy		Lower Hypertrophy	
Upper Strength	Lower Strength		Upper Hypertrophy		Lower Hypertrophy	
Upper Strength	Lower Strength		Upper Hypertrophy		Lower Hypertrophy	
Upper Strength	Lower Strength		Upper Hypertrophy		Lower Hypertrophy	

Upper Strength

Exercise	Sets	Reps	Rest (min)	Tempo
1: Barbell Bench Press	4-set method	4–6	3	4010
2: Chin-up	4-set method	4–6	3	4010
3: Barbell Military Press	4-set method	4–6	3	4010
4: Chest-Supported Row	4-set method	4–6	3	4010
5: Barbell Curl	4	6–8	2	3010
6: Lying Triceps Extension	4	6–8	2	3010

Lower Strength

Exercise	Sets	Reps	Rest (min)	Tempo
1: Squat or Bulgarian Split Squat	4-set method	4–6	3	4010
2: Rack Deadlift or Single-Leg Deadlift	4-set method	4–6	3	4010
3: Walking Lunges	4	6–8 each leg	3	4010
4: Hamstring Curls	4	6–8	3	4010
5: Standing Calf Raises	4	10–15	2	3010

Upper Hypertrophy

Exercise	Sets	Reps	Rest (min)	Tempo
1A: Barbell Military Press	4-set method	6–8	1.5	3010
1B: Chin-up	4-set method	6–8	1.5	3010
2A: Barbell Bench Press	4-set method	6–8	1.5	3010

2B: Chest-Supported Row	4-set method	6–8	1.5	3010
3A: Chest-Supported Dumbbell Lateral Raises	3	10–12	1	3010
3B: Incline Dumbbell Press	3	10–12	1	3010
3C: Seated Cable Row	3	10–12	1	3010
4A: Incline Dumbbell Curls	3	10–12	1	3010
4B: Rope Pulley Triceps Extension	3	10–12	1	3010

Lower Hypertrophy

Exercise	Sets	Reps	Rest (min)	Tempo
1: Hamstring Curls	3	8–12	1	3010
2: Squat or Bulgarian Split Squat	4-set method	6–8	1.5	3010
3: Rack Deadlift or Single-Leg Deadlift	4-set method	6–8	1.5	3010
4: Walking Lunges or Hack Squat or Smith Machine Squat	3	20–25	3	3010
5: Calf Raises	4	15-25	1.5	3010

Chapter 18:
Advanced Strength and Mass

You are considered advanced after you've lifted for more than four years, have attained the strong levels cited in the "How Strong Is Strong Enough? chapter, and have made great progress with your body. Your goal now is to move from strong to the aesthetically strong levels below.

Exercise	Strength Goal (1RM)
Bench Press	1.5 x body weight
Single-Arm Bench Press	0.6 x body weight
Weighted Chin-up	0.75 x body weight
Barbell Military Press	1 x body weight
Single-Arm Dumbbell Military Press	0.4 x body weight
Back Squat	2 x body weight
Bulgarian Split Squat	1.2 x body weight
Deadlift	2.5 x body weight
Single-Leg Deadlift	1.65 x body weight

To summarize, continue with the advanced strength and mass phase until you reach the aesthetically strong goals in the table above. Make sure to follow "The Plan" chapter for an overview of your *Muscle* journey.

Advanced Strength and Mass Key Features

- Get strong first
- Build dense muscle

- Do 3–4 days per week
- Lengthen rest periods the heavier the weight
- Use these workouts to become aesthetically strong
- Gain your next 5–10 lb. (2–5 kg) of muscle (you're advanced after all)

The 4-Set Method

The advanced strength and mass phase continues using the 4-set method introduced in the intermediate strength and mass phase.

Let's Train All the Time Baby

At the advanced level, the weights you lift will be heavy. Long workouts will be a thing of the past, as they will leave you drained and affect your recovery. This is why most advanced bodybuilders do bro splits, which allow them to work a muscle group intensely and then let it recover for a week.

Bro splits do work for advanced trainees. But I don't believe them to be the best way to train. Instead of training each body part once a week, it is better to spread the workout volume across a six-day schedule. You still train each body part twice a week, but you are spreading intensity throughout the week and thereby facilitating recovery.

Advanced Strength and Mass Schedule

Your workout schedule utilizes a six-day split of push, pull, legs for strength and of push, pull, legs for hypertrophy as follows:

6 Days per Week

Sunday	Monday	Tuesday	Wednesday	Thursday	Friday	Saturday
	Push (Strength)	Pull (Strength)	Legs (Strength)	Push (Hypertrophy)	Pull (Hypertrophy)	Legs (Hypertrophy)
	Push (Strength)	Pull (Strength)	Legs (Strength)	Push (Hypertrophy)	Pull (Hypertrophy)	Legs (Hypertrophy)
	Push (Strength)	Pull (Strength)	Legs (Strength)	Push (Hypertrophy)	Pull (Hypertrophy)	Legs (Hypertrophy)
	Push (Strength)	Pull (Strength)	Legs (Strength)	Push (Hypertrophy)	Pull (Hypertrophy)	Legs (Hypertrophy)

Push (Strength)

Exercise	Sets	Reps	Rest (min)	Tempo
1: Barbell Bench Press	4-set method	4–6	3	4010
2: Barbell Military Press	4-set method	4–6	3	4010
3: Dumbbell Bench Press	4-set method	4–6	3	4010
4: Cable Triceps Press down	3–4	8–10	2	3010

Pull (Strength)

Exercise	Sets	Reps	Rest (min)	Tempo
1: Chest-Supported Dumbbell Row	4-set method	4–6	3	4010
2: Weighted Chin-ups	4-set method	4–6	3	4010
3: Barbell Bent Over Row	4-set method	4–6	3	4010
4: Biceps Curls	3	10–12	2	3010

Legs (Strength)

Exercise	Sets	Reps	Rest (min)	Tempo
1: Squat or Bulgarian Split Squat	4-set method	4–6	3	4010
2: Rack or Single-Leg Deadlift	4-set method	4–6	3	4010
3: Walking Lunges	4	6–8 each leg	3	4010
4: Hamstring Curls	4	6–8	3	4010
5: Standing Calf Raises	4	10–15	2	3010

Push (Hypertrophy)

Exercise	Sets	Reps	Rest (min)	Tempo
1: Low-Incline Dumbbell Bench Press	4-set method	6–8	3	4010
2: Dumbbell Military Press	4-set method	6–8	3	4010
3: Close-Grip Bench Press	4-set method	6–8	3	4010

4: Dumbbell Flys	4	10–12	2	3010
5: Dumbbell Lateral Raise	3	12–15	2	3010

Pull (Hypertrophy)

Exercise	Sets	Reps	Rest (min)	Tempo
1: Single-Arm Dumbbell Row	4-set method	6–8	3	4010
2: Lat Pull down	4-set method	6–8	3	4010
3: Hang & Swings	3	30	2	3010
4: Biceps Curls	3	12–15	2	3010

Legs (Hypertrophy)

Exercise	Sets	Reps	Rest (min)	Tempo
1: Hamstring Curls	3	8–12	1	3010
2: Squat or Bulgarian Split Squat	4-set method	6–8	1.5	3010
3: Rack or Single-Leg Dead-lift	4-set method	6–8	1.5	3010
4: Walking Lunges or Hack Squat or Smith Ma-chine Squat	3	20–25	3	3010
5: Calf Raises	4	15–25	1.5	3010

Chapter 19:
Specialization

Professional arm wrestlers are an example of specialization. Each has an enormous dominant upper limb whose forearm, biceps, and triceps can be several times larger than on the opposite arm. Google Matthias Schlitte, and you'll see what I mean. Train a specific body part repeatedly to the neglect of other parts, and the trained part will grow disproportionately.

In the chapter "Steve Reeves's Secret to Head-on Collisions," I discussed perfect proportions. This is your aim after you've built a foundation of strength and muscle over a year or two of advanced training. It's time to precisely chisel your body by specializing, not to overemphasize parts at the expense of others but, rather, to make lagging parts proportional.

Which Body Parts Need Specialization?

Look in a mirror. Which body part looks smaller than others, your legs, arms, chest, back? A lagging body part will stick out like a sore thumb. If you don't notice obvious weaknesses, check to see how close your body measurements are to the ideal proportions defined earlier in this book. A significant difference points to a need to specialize on the smaller body part. You can also check your strength levels against those in the "How Strong Is Strong Enough" chapter. Weakness in a lift indicates your need to specialize on the body part affected by that lift.

The absence of weaknesses, conversely, indicates that you don't need to specialize. You can continue to do strength and hypertrophy workouts or you can specialize just for fun.

How the Specialization Programs Work

This chapter offers a specialization program of 4–8 weeks for each major body part. You will then move to strength or hypertrophy workouts from the appropriate chapters.

Every specialization program trains its specific body part at high volume and frequency, with lots of sets and reps 3–4 days a week. The goal is to stimulate the muscle every 48–72 hours. This maximizes protein synthesis and provides ample mechanical tension, metabolic stress, and muscle damage—the mechanisms of muscle growth.

Upon completing a specialization program, you might notice zero growth in the target body part. Yes, you read that correctly: zero. This is because you will overreach the muscle by the end of the program. At this point, you will return to strength or hypertrophy workouts. A week or so later, you will notice the supercompensation of the specialized body part. This is when growth occurs. By dialing back the training of that body part, the muscle speeds its recovery, and quick muscle growth results. Think of it like muscle-building momentum.

Specialization Program Schedule

Sunday	Monday	Tuesday	Wednesday	Thursday	Friday	Saturday
Workout A	Workout B		Workout C		Workout D	Optional Workout
Workout A	Workout B		Workout C		Workout D	Optional Workout

Arm Specialization

Workout A

Exercise	Sets	Reps	Rest (min)	Tempo
1: Front or Bulgarian Split Squat	3	10–12 each leg	2	3010
2: Chest-Supported Row or Chin-up	3	8–12	2	3010
3: Rack or Single-Leg Deadlift	3	8–12	2	3010
4: Dumbbell Bench Press	3	8–12	2	3010

5: Dumbbell Overhead Press	3	8–12	2	3010

Workout B

Exercise	Sets	Reps	Rest (min)	Tempo
1: Weighted Close-Grip Chin-ups	5	5–8	3	4010
2: Close-Grip Bench Press	5	5–8	3	4010
3A: Cable Biceps Curl	3–4	6–8 + rest pause on last set*	2	4010
3B: Cable Triceps Press down	3–4	6–8 + rest pause on last set*	2	4010

*Rest for 15 seconds and then do as many reps as possible at the same weight. Rest another 15 seconds and again do as many reps as possible.

Workout C

Exercise	Sets	Reps	Rest (min)	Tempo
1: Weighted Close-Grip Chin-ups	4	8–12	3	3010
2: Close-Grip Bench Press	4	8–12	3	3010
3: Incline Dumbbell Curls	2–3	8–12 + quadruple drop set on last set*	2	3010
4: Lying Triceps Extension	2–3	8–12 + quadruple drop set on last set*	2	3010

*After the last set, immediately reduce the weight 15–30% and do as many reps as possible. Repeat four times.

Workout D

Exercise	Sets	Reps	Rest (min)	Tempo
1: Weighted Close-Grip Chin-ups	3	12–15	3	2010
2: Close-Grip Bench Press	3	12–15	3	2010
3: Dumbbell Hammer Curls	2–3	8–12 + quadruple drop set on last set*	2	2010
4: Lying Triceps Extension	2–3	8–12 + quadruple drop set on last set*	2	2010

*After the last set, immediately reduce the weight 15–30% and do as many reps as possible. Repeat four times.

Optional Workout

Exercise	Sets	Reps	Rest (min)	Tempo
1: Barbell Curl	As few as possible (ALAP)*	100 total reps	1	2010
2: Cable Triceps Pressdown	ALAP	100 total reps	1	2010

*The optional workout infuses the target body part with blood. Do a set of as many reps as possible using a light weight easily handled for 20–25 reps. Rest 1 minute and repeat. Rest another minute and repeat until you reach 100 total reps.

Chest Specialization

Workout A

Exercise	Sets	Reps	Rest (min)	Tempo
1: Front or Bulgarian Split Squat	3	10–12 each leg	2	3010
2: Chest-Supported Row or Chin-up	3	8–12	2	3010
3: Rack or Single-Leg Deadlift	3	8–12	2	3010
4: Dumbbell Overhead Press	3	8–12	2	3010
5A: Dumbbell Curls	3	8–12	2	3010
5B: Cable Triceps Extensions	3	8–12	2	3010

Workout B

Exercise	Sets	Reps	Rest (min)	Tempo
1: Barbell Bench Press	5	5–8	3	4010
2: Incline Dumbbell Bench Press	4	5–8	3	4010
3: Weighted Push-ups	3–4	6–8 + rest pause on last set*	2	4010
4: Batwing Rows	3–4	10	2	4010

*Rest for 15 seconds and then do as many reps as possible at the same weight. Rest another 15 seconds and again do as many reps as possible.

Workout C

Exercise	Sets	Reps	Rest (min)	Tempo
1: Barbell Bench Press	4	8–12	3	3010
2: Cable Chest Press	3	8–12	3	3010
3: Incline Dumbbell Bench Press	2–3	8–12 + quadruple drop set on last set*	2	3010
4: Seated Cable Row	2–3	8–12	2	3010

*After the last set, immediately reduce the weight 15–30% and do as many reps as possible. Repeat four times.

Workout D

Exercise	Sets	Reps	Rest (min)	Tempo
1: Incline Barbell Bench Press	3	12–15	3	2010
2: Weighted Push-ups	3	12–15	3	2010
3: Flat Dumbbell Bench Press	2–3	8–12 + quadruple drop set on last set*	2	2010
4: Inverted Rows	2–3	8–12	2	2010

*After the last set, immediately reduce the weight 15–30% and do as many reps as possible. Repeat four times.

Optional Workout

Exercise	Sets	Reps	Rest (min)	Tempo
1: Push-ups	As few as possible (ALAP)*	150 total reps	1	2010

*The optional workout infuses the target body part with blood. Do a set of as many reps as possible. Rest 1 minute and repeat. Rest another minute and repeat to reach 150 total reps.

Back Specialization

Workout A

Exercise	Sets	Reps	Rest (min)	Tempo
1: Front or Bulgarian Split Squat	3	10–12 each leg	2	3010
2: Barbell Bench Press	3	8–12	2	3010
3: Rack or Single-Leg Deadlift	3	8–12	2	3010
4: Dumbbell Overhead Press	3	8–12	2	3010
5A: Dumbbell Curls	3	8–12	2	3010
5B: Cable Triceps Extensions	3	8–12	2	3010

Workout B

Exercise	Sets	Reps	Rest (min)	Tempo
1: Weighted Chin-ups	5	5–8	3	4010
2: Chest-Supported Row	5	5–8	3	4010
3: Chest-Supported Row (yes, this is not a typo)	4	6–8 + rest pause on last set*	2	4010

*Rest for 15 seconds and then do as many reps as possible at the same weight. Rest another 15 seconds and again do as many reps as possible.

Workout C

Exercise	Sets	Reps	Rest (min)	Tempo
1: Chest-Supported Row	4	8–12	3	3010
2: Lat Pull down	4	8–12	3	3010
3: Cable Pullover	3	8–12 + quadruple drop set on last set*	2	3010

*After the last set, immediately reduce the weight 15–30% and do as many reps as possible. Repeat four times.

Workout D

Exercise	Sets	Reps	Rest (min)	Tempo
1: Chest-Supported Row	3	12–15	3	2010
2: Gironda Lat Pull	3	12–15	3	2010

3: Lat Pull downs	3	8–12 + quadruple drop set on last set*	2	2010

Optional Workout

Exercise	Sets	Reps	Rest (min)	Tempo
1: Chin-ups	As few as possible (ALAP)*	50 total reps	1	2010

*The optional workout infuses the target body part with blood. Do a set of as many reps as possible. Rest 1 minute and repeat. Rest another minute and repeat to reach 50 total reps.

Shoulder Specialization

Workout A

Exercise	Sets	Reps	Rest (min)	Tempo
1: Front or Bulgarian Split Squat	3	10–12 each leg	2	3010
2: Chest-Supported Row or Chin-up	3	8–12	2	3010
3: Rack or Single-Leg Deadlift	3	8–12	2	3010
4: Barbell Bench Press	3	8–12	2	3010
5A: Dumbbell Curls	3	8–12	2	3010
5B: Cable Triceps Extensions	3	8–12	2	3010

Workout B

Exercise	Sets	Reps	Rest (min)	Tempo
1: Barbell Military Press	5	5–8	3	4010
2: Single-Arm Dumbbell Overhead Press	4	5–8	3	4010
3: Dumbbell Lateral Raises	3–4	6–8 + rest pause on last set*	2	4010
4: Batwing Rows	3–4	10	2	4010

*Rest for 15 seconds and then do as many reps as possible at the same weight. Rest another 15 seconds and again do as many reps as possible.

Workout C

Exercise	Sets	Reps	Rest (min)	Tempo
1: Barbell Military Press	4	8–12	3	3010
2: Chest Supported Reverse Dumbbell Flyes	3	8–12	3	3010
3: Chest-Supported Lateral Raises (80–85° incline)	2–3	8–12 + quadruple drop set on last set*	2	3010
4: Seated Cable Row	2–3	8–12	2	3010

*After the last set, immediately reduce the weight 15–30% and do as many reps as possible. Repeat four times.

Workout D

Exercise	Sets	Reps	Rest (min)	Tempo
1: Cable Lateral Raises	3	12–15	3	2010
2: Chest-Supported Reverse Flys	3	12–15	3	2010
3: Dumbbell Overhead Press	2–3	8–12 + quadruple drop set on last set*	2	2010
4: Inverted Rows	2–3	8–12	2	2010

*After the last set, immediately reduce the weight 15–30% and do as many reps as possible. Repeat four times.

Optional Workout

Exercise	Sets	Reps	Rest (min)	Tempo
1: Lateral Raises	As few as possible (ALAP)*	150 total reps	1	2010

*The optional workout infuses the target body part with blood. Do a set of as many reps as possible using a light weight easily handled for 20–25 reps. Rest 1 minute and repeat. Rest another minute and repeat until you reach 150 total reps.

Leg Specialization

Workout A

Exercise	Sets	Reps	Rest (min)	Tempo
1: Dumbbell Curls	3	10–12 each leg	2	3010
2: Chest-Supported Row or Chin-up	3	8–12	2	3010
3: Cable Triceps Press down	3	8–12	2	3010
4: Dumbbell Bench Press	3	8–12	2	3010
5: Dumbbell Overhead Press	3	8–12	2	3010

Workout B

Exercise	Sets	Reps	Rest (min)	Tempo
1: Hamstring Curls	5	5–8	3	4010
2: Bulgarian Split Squat	5	5-8	3	4010
3A: Rack Deadlift	3–4	6–8 + rest pause on last set*	2	4010
3B: Front Squats	3–4	6–8 + rest pause on last set*	2	4010

*Rest for 15 seconds and then do as many reps as possible at the same weight. Rest another 15 seconds and again do as many reps as possible.

Workout C

Exercise	Sets	Reps	Rest (min)	Tempo
1: Hamstring Curls	4	8–12+ quadruple drop set on last set*	3	3010
2: Back or Front Squats	4	8–12 + quadruple drop set on last set*	3	3010
3: Walking Lunges	2–3	8–12	2	3010
4: Romanian Deadlift	2–3	8–12	2	3010

*After the last set, immediately reduce the weight 15–30% and do as many reps as possible. Repeat four times.

Workout D

Exercise	Sets	Reps	Rest (min)	Tempo
1: Hamstring Curls	3	12–15 + quadruple drop set on last set*	3	2010
2: Bulgarian Split Squat	3	12–15	3	2010
3: Front or Back Squat	2–3	8–12 + quadruple drop set on last set*	2	2010
4: Rack Deadlift	2–3	8–12	2	2010

Optional Workout

Exercise	Sets	Reps	Rest (min)	Tempo
1: Hamstring Curls	As few as possible (ALAP)*	100 total reps	1	2010
2: Back Squats	ALAP	100 total reps	1	2010

*The optional workout infuses the target body part with blood. Do a set of as many reps as possible using a light weight easily handled for 20–25 reps. Rest 1 minute and repeat. Rest another minute and repeat until you reach 100 total reps.

Chapter 20:
Maintenance

Imagine having the perfect body. You look in the mirror and are 100% happy with what you see. You are lean but hugely muscular and very strong. How should you continue training?

Many people think that once they reach their muscle-building goal they can stop training. They tell themselves, "if I can gain 30 lb. (14 kg) of muscle and lose 20 lb. (9 kg) of fat, I can cancel my gym membership and eat what I want, and I'll look the same." Anyone who's ever been incapacitated by injury knows this is wrong. Stop training, and you'll lose the body that you worked so hard to achieve.

Your dream body needs maintaining. You won't have to work as hard as you did to achieve it, but you do need to put in some effort to maintain it.

How to Maintain Your Dream Physique

Maintenance is a lot simpler than you might think. Training once a week preserves muscle strength. Another once-weekly session, of hypertrophy work, protects muscle size. So your training volume can be low, and you can get away with training several times a week.

You can't, however, slack off in the gym training for maintenance. You still need to push yourself to get stronger with each exercise. This ensures that you don't lose muscle and that you burn enough calories to stoke your metabolism and stay lean. High strength and muscle mass will allow you to eat more daily without unwanted weight gains.

I've found the following the best method for maintenance:

- Train 2–3 times a week, with at least one full-body session once a week.
- Take long rest periods (3 minutes for compound lifts, and 2 for non-compound lifts).
- Use reverse pyramid training (RPT) to maintain and gain strength.
- Use RPT rest pause training to maintain muscle size.

Your maintenance workouts are based on the minimalist approach long advocated by such fitness professionals as Greg O'Gallagher and Martin Berkhan.

2-Days-per-Week Maintenance Schedule

Sun-day	Monday	Tues-day	Wednes-day	Thurs-day	Fri-day	Satur-day
	Workout A			Workout B		
	Workout A			Workout B		

2-Days-per-Week Maintenance Workout A

Exercise	Sets	Reps	Rest (min)	Tempo
1A: Barbell Bench Press	3 (RPT)	4–6, 6–8, 8–10	3	3010
1B: Chest-Supported Row	3 (RPT)	4–6, 6–8, 8–10	3	3010
2A: Dumbbell or Barbell Military Press	3 (RPT)	4–6, 6–8, 8–10	3	3010
2B: Chin-up or Lat Pull down	3 (RPT)	4–6, 6–8, 8–10	3	3010
3: Incline Dumbbell Bench Press	RPT rest pause	12–15, then 4 sets of 3–5	2 (after completing full rest pause set)	2010
4: Seated Cable Row	RPT rest pause	12–15, then 4 sets of 3–5	2 (after completing full rest pause set)	2010
5: Dumbbell Lateral Raises	RPT rest pause	12–15, then 4 sets of 3–5	2 (after completing full rest pause set)	2010

2-Days-per-Week Maintenance Workout B

Exercise	Sets	Reps	Rest (min)	Tempo
1: Rack Dead-lift	3 (RPT)	4–6, 6–8, 8–10	3	3010
2: Squats or Bulgarian Split Squats	3 (RPT)	4–6, 6–8, 8–10	3	3010
3: Walking Lunges	RPT rest pause	12–15, then 4 sets of 3–5	2 (after completing full rest pause set)	2010
4: Calf Raises	RPT rest pause	12–15, then 4 sets of 3–5	2 (after completing full rest pause set)	2010
5: Incline Dumbbell Curl	RPT rest pause	12–15, then 4 sets of 3-5	2 (after completing full rest pause set)	2010
6: Lying Triceps Extension	RPT rest pause	12–15, then 4 sets of 3–5	2 (after completing full rest pause set)	2010

3-Days-per-Week Maintenance Schedule

Sunday	Monday	Tuesday	Wednesday	Thursday	Friday	Saturday
	Workout A		Workout B		Workout C	
	Workout A		Workout B		Workout C	

3-Days-per-Week Maintenance Workout A

Exercise	Sets	Reps	Rest (min)	Tempo
1: Bench Press (Barbell or Dumbbell)	3 (RPT)	4–6, 6–8, 8–10	3	3010
2: Barbell Military Press or Single-Arm	3 (RPT)	4–6, 6–8, 8–10	3	3010

Dumbbell Military Press				
3: Lying Triceps Extension	3 (RPT)	4–6, 6–8, 8–10	2	3010
4: Incline Dumbbell Bench Press	RPT rest pause	12–15, then 4 sets of 3–5	2 (after completing full rest pause set)	2010
5: Dumbbell Lateral Raises	RPT rest pause	12–15, then 4 sets of 3–5	2 (after completing full rest pause set)	2010
6: Rope Triceps Press down	RPT rest pause	12–15, then 4 sets of 3–5	2 (after completing full rest pause set)	2010

3-Days-per-Week Maintenance Workout B

Exercise	Sets	Reps	Rest (min)	Tempo
1: Chin-ups (Use weight if necessary)	3 (RPT)	4–6, 6–8, 8–10	3	3010
2: Chest-Supported Dumbbell Row	3 (RPT)	4–6, 6–8, 8–10	3	3010
3: Barbell Curl	3 (RPT)	4–6, 6–8, 8–10	2	3010
4: Lat Pull down	RPT rest pause	12–15, then 4 sets of 3–5	2 (after completing full rest pause set)	2010
5: Seated Cable Row	RPT rest pause	12–15, then 4 sets of 3–5	2 (after completing full rest pause set)	2010
6: Incline Dumbbell Curl	RPT rest pause	12–15, then 4 sets of 3-5	2 (after completing full rest pause set)	2010

3-Days-per-Week Maintenance Workout C

Exercise	Sets	Reps	Rest (min)	Tempo
1: Squat or Bulgarian Split Squat	3 (RPT)	4–6, 6–8, 8–10	3	3010
2: Rack Dead-lift	3 (RPT)	4–6, 6–8, 8–10	3	3010
3: Walking Lunges	RPT rest pause	12–15, then 4 sets of 3–5	2 (after completing full rest pause set)	2010
4: Leg Curls	RPT rest pause	12–15, then 4 sets of 3–5	2 (after completing full rest pause set)	2010
5: Calf Raises	RPT rest pause	12–15, then 4 sets of 3–5	2 (after completing full rest pause set)	2010

When to Use Maintenance Workouts

Maintenance workouts are to be performed once you've reached your muscle-building goal. They are minimalist sessions designed to maintain your muscle strength and mass without requiring hour after hour week in the gym.

I recommend doing maintenance workouts for as many as eight months consecutively before moving on to 12 weeks of the base building that you need to do yearly. Following the base-building work, perform workouts of your choosing for a month from among the specialization, hypertrophy, and strength workouts. It doesn't matter which; it's up to you.

Chapter 21:
Recovery: Your Natural Steroid

We've all experienced it. You have a great leg workout where you push your body to its limit, chasing the pump by doing set after set. Drop sets. Rest pauses. Forced reps. You do them all.

The next day, you wake up, get out of bed, and you can barely walk. It's almost as if your legs aged 60 years overnight. The next few days, you have trouble doing the simple things in life, like walking to the corner store, climbing stairs, and sitting on the toilet. What went wrong?

A lot of guys think that if they have the perfect workout in the gym, things will take care of themselves afterward. "Bro, I'll just get a crazy good pump, and then I'll get bigger. I don't focus on nutrition, stretching, sleep, and supplements. All you need is hard work." The truth is, the workout is half the battle. The other half is making sure that your recovery is fantastic.

Optimizing your recovery will optimize your muscle growth. You need to focus on three things in this order of importance: sleep, nutrition and supplements, and movement quality.

Sleep

I'm just going to say it. Sleep is the most anabolic activity you can do, more than lifting weights, more than eating lots of protein. Sleep provides what your body needs: ample rest and regeneration.

Think about the last time you had a long, deep sleep. How did you feel afterwards? You woke up feeling refreshed and relaxed. Your body felt good. Your mind felt good. If you trained that day, you would have noticed that you were able to focus better and possibly lift heavier. Imagine what would happen if you had a long and deep sleep every single night.

Sleep not only leaves you refreshed and focused, it also increases your growth hormone and testosterone levels. Instead of taking low doses of steroids, many guys could be getting similar results from improved sleep. A 2007 study showed that men who slept 8 or more hours a night had double the testosterone levels of men who slept only 4 hours a night. The bottom line: aim for 8 hours of sleep per night.

How to Optimize Sleep

Optimizing your sleep takes more than simply saying, "tonight I'm going to get 8 hours of sleep." There are too many variables. What if you toss and turn and have trouble falling asleep? What if you wake up to use the bathroom? What if you can't fall back asleep? You need to make getting a good night's sleep a habit by teaching your internal clock to recognize a certain period as your time for sleep. I recommend doing the following:

Create a Sleep Schedule

The best way to have long, peaceful sleeps is to go to bed at the same time every night and to wake up at the same time every morning. If you wake at 6 a.m., you need to be asleep by 10 p.m. Using the technique I'm about to teach you, it'll take 10–30 minutes to fall sleep, so 9:30 p.m. should be lights out. Once you determine these parameters, you need to follow them religiously for two consecutive weeks to make them a habit.

Your Room and the BSDQT Formula

The sleep schedule you establish will help you sleep longer. The BSDQT formula—of bed, stress, dark, quiet, and temperature—will help you sleep deeper.

Your bed is among the most important investments you can make. If you sleep 8 hours a night, you're spending a third of your life in bed. So make sure you have a good one. Your mattress in particular should be of high quality. Tossing and turning all night is not natural.

If you've ever stayed in a nice hotel, you've probably noticed that you slept deeply. It's because quality hotels usually have quality mattresses. So save up for a great mattress, preferably a great box spring. Your bed should make you feel like a million bucks, should support your spine in perfect alignment, and should last at least 10 years to offset the investment.

When you go to bed, you need to be as free of stress as possible. Stress will prevent the length and the depth of your sleep. I've found that meditating after finishing work and reading fiction before bed help me reduce stress significantly.

You also want your room to be dark. Our bodies have evolved to produce melatonin—a hormone that regulates sleep and wake cycles—when it's dark. This is why we sleep at night. To darken your bedroom further, you might want to invest in blackout curtains. You'll also want to examine your bedroom for light from electronics, such as your alarm clock. Cover these lights at night. And avoid such as smartphones, laptops, and tablets before bed. The glow from their screens is known to suppress melatonin.

Quiet, too, is imperative for sound sleep. Noise makes it hard to fall and stay asleep. In the event of noise over which you have no control, such as the noisy neighbors in the apartment above mine in a building I once lived in, the solutions are white noise from a fan, for instance, or earplugs. I utilize both.

The temperature in your bedroom is likewise an issue for good sleep. A study from Canada's National Sleep Foundation found that we sleep best in a cool bedroom and recommends temperatures of 16–19° Celsius (61–66° Fahrenheit). I can attest to sleeping deeply within this temperature range. But adjust the temperature to suit yourself or use heavier or extra blankets. Being cold won't help you sleep.

Nutrition and Supplementation

What you eat will directly affect your muscles ability to recover. Training will inevitably break down muscle fiber. You need good nutrition to help repair the damage. I look in-depth at nutrition in part 3 of this book, but for now keep in mind this mantra: Meat for strength. Veggies for health. Carbohydrates for muscle.

Movement Quality

Professional ice hockey players typically do 15–20 minutes on a stationary bike the day after a game. This "flushes" the muscles and helps with soreness. The motion promotes blood circulation in the muscles, helping to transport in vital nutrients and to transport out the by-products of hard work. It's simply good practice to move your whole body as part of your recovery process. This could be as simple as foam rolling, doing the warm-up that you normally do before working out, stretching, hiking, swimming, or playing another sport. This is active recovery for bodies meant to move.

Reference

Penev, Plamen D. "Association Between Sleep and Morning Testosterone Levels In Older Men." *Sleep*, vol. 30, no. 4, 2007, pp. 427–432., doi:10.1093/sleep/30.4.427.

Chapter 22:
Exercise Descriptions

Back Squat

With a loaded barbell on your shoulders/top of back, squat down like you're taking a crap in the woods. Keep your knees wide. Go down until your thighs are just below parallel to the floor. Stand back up. Repeat.

Backward Crawl

Get on your hands and knees as if to crawl like a baby. Lift your knees off the ground so that you're on only your toes and hands. Crawl backward while keeping your spine straight. If you do this right, you'll feel it in your core muscles.

Barbell Bench Press

Lie down on the bench with your feet planted on the floor. Unrack the barbell and lower it to your chest. Press the bar upward until your arms are almost straight. Repeat.

Barbell Bent Over Row

Grasp a barbell with an overhand grip. Stand up straight, push your butt back, and slide the bar down your thighs until it touches your knees. This is your starting position. Forcefully push your elbows back until the bar touches your chest/stomach. Lower the bar back to the starting position under control. Repeat.

Barbell Curl

Hold a barbell with underhand grip, hands shoulder width apart. Keep your elbows at your sides and bend at the elbows by squeezing your biceps until your forearms are vertical. Lower the bar until your arms are straight. Repeat.

Barbell Military Press

Stand holding a barbell in front at shoulder height. Your hands and feet should be shoulder width apart. Press the barbell above your head, then lower it with control back down to your collar bone. Repeat.

Barbell Romanian Deadlift

Grasp a barbell with overhand grip, hands slightly wider than shoulders, and stand tall. Stand with your feet a bit narrower than shoulder width. Lower the bar by bending at the hips, bending slightly at the knees, and pushing your butt back. Keep your shins parallel to the floor, and slide the bar along the thighs throughout the movement. Lower the bar until it's below knee height. You should feel a stretch in the hamstrings. Squeeze your glutes and stand back up straight. Slide the bar up your thighs throughout the movement. Repeat.

Bulgarian Split Squat

Stand holding two dumbbells at your sides while facing away from a bench. Extend one leg back and place the top of the foot on the bench. Squat by bending your forward knee. Go down until your opposite, back knee almost touches the floor. Return to the original standing position by pushing through your heel. Do all reps for one leg and then move to the other for one set.

Cable Romanian Deadlift

Grasp a cable with the overhand grip, hands slightly wider than shoulders. The pulley should be as low as possible. Stand with feet a bit narrower than shoulder width. Bend at the hips and slightly at the knees and push your butt back. Keep your shins parallel to the floor throughout the movement. Lower the cable until it's at knee height. You should feel a stretch in the hamstrings. Squeeze your glutes and stand back up straight. Repeat.

Cable Triceps Press down/Push down

Face a high pulley and grasp the rope attachment with both hands. Put your elbows at your sides. Extend your arms downward, flexing the triceps, until your arms are extended. Bend at the elbows to bring your hands back to starting position.

Chest-Supported Dumbbell Lateral Raises

Set up an incline bench at about 80–85^0. Stand up straight, with your arms at your sides, and press your chest against the bench while holding a dumbbell in each hand. With slightly bent elbows, raise your hands out to the side so that your arms form a T with your body. Try to push your hands as far away from your body as possible. Lower the dumbbells with control to the starting position. Repeat.

Chest-Supported Dumbbell Row

Lie chest down on an incline bench, holding dumbbells in each hand. Flex your back muscles and pull (row) the dumbbells upward until your thumbs are almost touching your armpits. Return your arms to their fully extended starting position. Repeat.

Close-Grip Bench Press

Same as barbell bench press but with a shoulder-width grip to focus on the triceps.

Deadlift

Grasp a barbell with an overhand grip, hands slightly wider than shoulders. Stand with your feet a bit narrower than shoulder width. Lower the bar to the floor by bending at the hips, bending slightly at the knees, and pushing your butt back. Keep your shins parallel to the floor throughout the movement. You should feel a slight stretch in the hamstrings at the bottom position. Squeeze your glutes to stand back up straight. Slide bar along the front of the body throughout the movement. Repeat.

Dumbbell Bench Press

Lie face up on a bench, holding dumbbells near your shoulders or at either side of your chest. Keep your elbows below your wrists at all times and press the dumbbells upward until your arms are extended. Lower the weight to the sides of your upper chest until you feel a slight stretch. Repeat.

Dumbbell Biceps Curl

Grasp a dumbbell in each hand. Keep your elbows at your side, and bend at the elbows until your forearms are vertical by flexing the biceps. Lower the dumbbells until your arms are straight. Repeat.

Dumbbell Flys

Lie face up on a bench. Grasp a dumbbell in each hand and move them straight above your chest, arms fully extended. Open your arms as if from an embrace to effect a stretch in your pecs and then bring your arms together in a hugging motion. Repeat.

Dumbbell Lateral Raise

Stand up straight, arms at your sides, a dumbbell in each hand. With slightly bent elbows, raise your hands out to the side so that your arms form a T with your body. Try to push your hands as far away from your body as possible. Lower the dumbbells with control to your starting position. Repeat.

Dumbbell Military Press

Stand tall, with dumbbells positioned at the side of your shoulders, your elbows below your wrists, and your forearms perpendicular to the floor. Press the dumbbells upward until your arms are fully extended overhead. Lower the dumbbells with control to the starting position. Repeat.

Dumbbell Step-up

Grasp a dumbbell in each hand. Stand in front of a bench, with one foot on the bench. Press your front foot into the bench to step up on to the bench. Lower yourself back down with control and the same leg. Repeat for given number of reps and then switch legs.

Forward Crawl

Get on your hands and knees as if to crawl like a baby. Lift your knees off of the ground so that you're on only your toes and hands. Crawl forward while keeping your spine straight. If you do this right, you'll feel it in your core muscles.

Front Plank

Lie face down on the floor. Press your elbows and toes into the ground and stiffen and straighten your body as it rises off the floor. Hold this straight, stiff position for the given time.

Front Squat

Hold a loaded barbell in front of your body at shoulder height by crossing your arms and placing your hands on top of the barbell, with your upper arms parallel to floor. Squat as if to take a crap in the woods. Keep your knees wide. Go down until your thighs are just below parallel to the floor. Stand back up. Repeat.

Goblet Squat

Hold a dumbbell vertically by one end. Hug it tight against your chest, with your elbows pointing down. Lower your body into a squat until you touch the pointy part of your elbow to the meaty part of your knee. Return to a standing position. Repeat.

Hack Squat

Follow the instructions on the hack squat machine. If no hack squat machine, use a leg press.

Half-Kneeling Single-Arm Dumbbell Press

Kneel with one knee on the floor and the other knee up and forward, ensuring that both knees are at a 90^0 angle. Grasp a dumbbell with your left hand and bring it to shoulder level. Press it overhead, then return it to your shoulder. Repeat for the designated reps and then switch legs and arms.

Hamstring Curls

Use either a lying hamstring curl machine or a seated hamstring curl machine. Start out with your legs straight, stretching your hamstrings. Bring your heels to your butt and lower under control. Pump your hamstrings.

Hang and Swings

Set up a bench at a 30^0 incline. Lie face down on the bench, your feet on the floor. Make your body long and tall, with your legs straight. Hold a heavy dumbbell in each hand and let your arms hang straight down. Pull your hands apart while keeping your arms straight. Swing your hands back and forth as if flying like a bird, slowly and controlled. Done right, you'll feel an intense burn in the back of your shoulders.

Heavy Farmer Carry

Grasp a heavy dumbbell in each hand, stand tall, and walk.

Incline Dumbbell Bench Press

Lie face up on a bench inclined to about 45^0. Hold dumbbells near both shoulders or at either side of your chest, keeping your elbows below your wrists at all times. Press the dumbbells up until your arms are fully extended. Lower the dumbells to the sides of your upper chest until you feel a slight stretch. Repeat.

Incline Dumbbell Curls

Set up a bench to a 60^0 incline. Grasp a dumbbell in each hand, sit on the bench, and lie back. Keep your elbows at your sides and bend them by flexing your biceps until your forearms are vertical. Lower the dumbbells until your arms are straight. Repeat.

Lat Pull down

Grasp the cable bar with a shoulder-width grip. Make sure your thighs are under the supports. Pull the cable bar down using your lats until the bar touches your collar bone or upper chest. Return the cable bar until your arms are fully extended above your body. Keep your elbows below your wrists at all times. Repeat.

Leg Curls

See hamstring curls.

Low-Incline Dumbbell Bench Press

Same as incline dumbbell bench press but with bench set at a lower incline.

Lying Triceps Extension

Lie on your back on a bench and position the dumbbells so that they are overhead, with your arms extended. Lower the dumbbells by bending at the elbows until the dumbbells are at the sides of your head and your forearms are parallel to the floor. Extend your arms by flexing the triceps. Repeat.

Push-up

Place your hands shoulder width apart on the floor, arms extended; lower your body to the floor; and then push it back up to starting position. Maintain a rigid body throughout. Repeat.

Quadruped Pull down

Set a cable pulley at the bottom position. Get down on your hands and knees. Extend your right arm and grasp the handle on the cable. Your arms should be straight and there should be tension in the cable. Pull your elbows to the sides of your body, initiating with your back muscles. Return your arms to the starting position. This is one rep. Do all reps and then repeat with the left arm.

Quadruped Row

Get down on your hands and knees as if to crawl like a baby. With a dumbbell in your right hand, pull your right elbow back to row the dumbbell up to your body. Reverse the movement. This is one rep. Do all reps on the right side, then switch and do all reps on the left side.

Rack Deadlift

Grasp a barbell with an overhand grip, hands slightly more than shoulder width. Stand with feet a bit less than shoulder width apart. Lower the bar to a power rack set up at knee or shin height by bending at the hips and slightly at the knees and by pushing your butt back, sliding the bar down your legs and keeping your shins parallel to the floor throughout the movement. You should feel a slight stretch in the hamstrings at the bottom position. Squeeze your glutes to stand back up, sliding the bar up the legs throughout the movement. Repeat.

Rear Delt Flys

Lie face down on an incline bench, holding dumbbells in each hand, arms straight down. Raise your arms to the side like the wings on an airplane. Try to push your hands as far from your body as possible. Lower yours arms to the starting position. Repeat. (You won't be able to use a full range of motion if you do a high number of reps. This is fine. Push through the pain.)

Reverse Lunge

Stand tall, feet together, dumbbells in each hand. Take a big step back with one leg and lower its knee to the floor. Push through the floor with the heel of your front leg to come back to the starting position. Repeat.

Rope Pulley Triceps Extension

Face a high pulley and grasp the rope attachment with both hands, elbows at sides. Extend your arms down by flexing the triceps until your arms are straight. Bend at the elbows to bring hands back to starting position.

Seated Cable Row

Sit at a cable row station, back erect, and hold this position through the movement. Grasp the cable attachment with extended arms. Pull with your back muscles by driving your elbows behind your body. Push your chest out and keep pulling until the cable attachment touches your stomach. Extend your arms to return to the starting position. Keep your shoulders low and away from your ears throughout the movement. Repeat.

Seated Calf Raises

Follow instructions on the machine.

Side Plank

Lie on one side and place your forearm on the floor under your shoulder so that your forearm is perpendicular to your body. Place your upper leg directly on top of your lower leg. Raise your body upward with your forearm by straightening your knees and hips until your body is rigidly straight. Hold this position for the allotted time.

Single-Arm Bench Press

Same as regular dumbbell bench press but with a single dumbbell. Do all sets on one side and then repeat on the other.

Single-Arm Cable Row

Set up a cable pulley at chest height. Take the handle in your right hand and walk back until there is tension in the cable. Take one step back with your right leg. Row the cable to you by pulling your right elbow back behind your body. Do all reps on one side before switching to the other side. (The hand holding the cable is on the same side as the back leg.)

Single-Arm Dumbbell Military Press

Same as regular military press but with only a single dumbbell. Do all reps on one side before switching and repeating on the other.

Single-Arm Dumbbell Row

Bend at the hips and place one knee and the same-side hand on a flat bench. Keep your other foot on the floor beside the bench. Hold a dumbbell in your free hand, letting it hang straight toward the floor, with your elbow loose. Pull the weight toward your hip, keeping your elbow close to your side as you flex your back, bend your arm, and bring your shoulder upward. At the top of the movement, your elbow should be pointed toward the ceiling as you squeeze your shoulder blades together. Lower the dumbbell under control along the same path. Complete your reps for one side, then switch arms and do the same number of reps on the other side to complete a set.

Single-Arm Farmer Carry

Same as farmer carry but with only one dumbbell held at the side.

Single-Arm Lat Pull down

Same as lat pull down but using a single handle attachment. Do all reps on one side, then switch and do all reps on the other side.

Single-Leg Cable Romanian Deadlift

Set up a cable pulley at the bottom position. Hold the handle attachment with your right hand. Take a few steps back until there is tension in the cable. Bend at the hips and bring your right leg off the floor. In your end position, your body will form a straight line from right leg to right arm, while your left foot remains on the floor. You should feel a stretch in your left hamstring and glute. Squeeze your left glute to return to the starting position. Do all reps on one side and then repeat on the other side.

Single-Leg Romanian Deadlift

Same as single-leg cable Romanian deadlift but using a dumbbell instead of a cable attachment.

Smith Machine Squat

Same as squat (below) but using a Smith machine.

Split Squat

Same as Bulgarian split squat but both feet are on the floor.

Back Squat

With loaded barbell over shoulders/top of back, squat down like you're taking a crap in the woods. Keep knees wide. Go down until thighs are just below parallel to the floor. Stand back up. Repeat.

Standing Calf Raises

Follow the instructions on the machine.

Standing Dumbbell Press

Same as dumbbell military press.

Walking Lunges

Take a large step forward. Bend both knees and bring your back knee to the floor. Press through the floor with the heel of the front leg and bring your back foot up to your front foot. Repeat on the other side.

Weighted Chin-ups

Grasp a pull-up bar with an underhand grip, shoulder width apart. Pull your body up until your chin reaches the bar. Keep your elbows at your sides. Lower your body until your arms are fully extended. Repeat.

SECTION 3:
EAT LIKE A KING

Chapter 23:
What's the Best Diet?

What's best, a low-carb, Paleo, Atkins, zone, vegetarian, vegan, or raw food diet or none of these? In truth, the best diet must do two things for you:

1. Achieve your desired results.
2. Be something that you can adhere to rigorously.

Because you want to build a lean, jacked physique, your diet must support minimal fat gain and maximum muscle growth. It should supply high levels of protein to fuel muscle development and help you recover from workouts.

But you've got to be able to stick with it. The best diet in the world yields no gains if you can't adhere to it. And this is where things get interesting. Dealing with daily issues can make following a strict diet tough. Your diet, therefore, needs to be flexible. Does this mean eating as much as you want, whatever you want, whenever you want? No. A flexible diet offers some leeway, but within reason.

Flexible Dieting 101

A flexible diet has minimum rules leading to maximum results. For fitness buffs, the essential, results-getting rules can be boiled down to the following:

1. A daily calorie requirement. Calories grant the energy your body needs. Eat as many calories as you burn, and you won't gain weight. Eat fewer calories than you burn, and you'll lose weight. Eat more calories than you burn, and you'll gain weight, either in muscle or fat. Calorie requirements vary by person. You'll learn to calculate your calorie requirement in the next chapter.

2. A daily protein requirement. Proteins build muscle, but how much protein you need varies by person. You will learn to calculate your protein requirement in the next chapter.

3. A daily vegetable requirement. Vegetables provide fiber and micronutrients essential for health. If you don't feel good, it's difficult to want to change your body. Get a minimum of 3 cups (710 ml) of non-starchy vegetables daily (you'll learn what these are shortly).

4. A daily water requirement. You do not need to drink 8 cups (1,893 ml) of water a day. Water requirements differ for individuals and depend on room temperature, respiration, etc. Drink sufficient water to ensure at least two clear urinations per day.

5. A daily meal requirement. Eat 2–6 meals daily for muscle building and 1–6 meals daily for fat loss.

6. A jacked-food requirement. Eat jacked foods 60–80% of the time (you'll find a list shortly).

You can see that these rules are pretty simple. Consume sufficient protein, calories, vegetables, and water daily, and you'll get the results you want. You don't even need set mealtimes. Just eat frequently throughout the day. Flexible dieting is pretty much free range. Want a doughnut for breakfast, a couple beers after work? Go ahead. Just make sure that your intake of jacked foods meets your daily requirements. I like flexible dieting because you can consume what you want as long as you don't break the six rules above.

A Note on Intermittent Fasting

Intermittent fasting is skipping breakfast and not eating during the first half of the day. Is breakfast the most important meal? It depends. Some people need breakfast, others don't. If you're skinny, chances are that skipping breakfast isn't the reason you can't build muscle. You'll get results hitting your macros—your total calorie and protein requirements—not focusing on eating breakfast or a lot. Flexible dieting permits you to skip a meal.

I intermittently fast daily because I like big meals. They leave me satisfied. I was a chubby child, so I think it's my inner fat kid who loves to eat lots at one meal. I typically don't eat until about 1 or 2 p.m. every day. Thereafter, I eat several large meals. Instead of spreading my daily calorie intake over a full day, I condense it into an 8–10-hour window. This is a great approach to dieting for fat loss, as you're dieting the first half of the day and eating normally thereafter.

Your diet is flexible. Don't force yourself to eat breakfast. And if you're busy at work and miss lunch, don't stress. Worrying about missing a meal is worse than missing the meal.

The Jacked Foods List

Following is a list of macro-friendly foods that should constitute 60–80% of your diet. The other 20–40% of your diet can come from eating whatever you want. This is the beauty of flexible dieting. You can eat what you want, get the results you want, and not have to feel guilty.

Proteins

- Meat, including poultry
- Wild game meat, including fowl and poultry
- Fish and seafood
- Eggs
- Protein powders with no fillers
- Cottage cheese (plain)
- Greek yogurt (plain)

Fats

- Fish oil
- Coconut oil
- Extra virgin olive oil
- Avocados
- Nuts and seeds
- Butter
- Meat fat

Carbohydrates

- Potatoes

- Sweet potatoes
- White rice
- Pumpkin
- Ezekiel bread
- Quinoa
- Wild rice
- All fruits
- Tubers
- Other grains
- Beans

Non-starchy Vegetables

Any vegetable that is not in the carbohydrate list above is considered non-starchy. This includes leafy greens, tomatoes, cucumbers, broccoli, cauliflower, etc.

Making Flexible Dieting Work for You

After calculating your daily calorie and protein requirements, which you'll learn how to do in the next chapter, you'll know how much you should eat per day. Then you have only to track what you eat to ensure that every day you hit those requirements. This seems like a big chore, but after tracking your intake for a couple of weeks it'll be second nature. Tracking your food intake can be done with a smartphone app, such as MyFitnessPal; with software available on the Internet, or with a spreadsheet.

Now start eating. My strategy is to eat from of the jacked foods list for the first half of the day, unless I'm meeting someone for breakfast or lunch. I like consuming large amounts of protein and vegetable at each meal. Mealtime examples include

- Large vegetable omelet
- Grilled meat with a side salad
- Roast chicken leg and roasted carrots

The evening is my favorite time to eat foods not on the jacked foods list. I know that if I eat most of my meals from that list, I'll nearly fulfill my protein and vegetable and calorie requirements. With sufficient calories during the day, I'm free to indulge later in pizza, fast food, ice cream, etc. I just need to know each evening how much junk food I can eat.

Some days, life gets in the way of a diet. There are surprise breakfasts or lunches with friends and family and the occasional too-tempting baked goods. When this happens, I'll usually eat what's on offer and not spurn it the way most diets advocate. I'll track it as part of my daily caloric intake. This means that I might not be able to fit additional junk food into my diet.

You don't, of course, have to eat junk food just because the diet is flexible. If you love eating healthy, by all means eat from the jacked foods list 100% of the time.

I simply want you to know that if you want something, you can have it. Listen to your body to figure out what it wants, then treat yourself.

Chapter 24:
Protein, Carbs, and Fat. Oh My!

This section of the book is about finding the optimal amounts of food to eat daily to reach your outcome goal. Breaking your intake into simple numbers of calories and grams of macronutrients eases the task of tracking your intake. If you're not getting the results you desire, you have only to look at your dietary figures and adjust accordingly.

Our Focus: Proteins and Calories

The calculations you'll learn focus on proteins and calories. Proteins are hands down the most important macronutrient for building and repairing muscle and are particularly effective in combination with a resistance training program. Calories are simply a unit of energy. Building muscle takes energy. You must eat a higher number of calories than you burn.

Why not eat as much as possible if calories help build muscle? Because muscle growth has a maximum speed. The key is to eat the correct number of calories to fuel the maximum speed of muscle growth. Excess calories end up as fat. You don't want this.

Imagine a slightly leaky bucket that you fill with water at a constant rate. The bucket represents how fast you can build muscle, and the water represents the calories needed for muscle growth at maximum speed. Fill the bucket too slowly, and it never fills up—the equivalent of not eating enough to build muscle. Fill the bucket too quickly, and it overflows—the equivalent of eating excessively and gaining fat.

Each year you train, moreover, the bucket gets smaller because the longer you train, the slower your muscle gain. You'll need, in other words, less food as an advanced trainee of five or more years than as a beginner trainee.

Where, meanwhile, do fats and carbohydrates fit in? The focus on calories and proteins does not imply eating steak only. Fulfill your calculated calorie and protein requirements, and you can be liberal in your daily carb and fat intake. It won't matter if you eat a high fat/low carb, low fat/high carb, or moderate fat/moderate carb diet provided you hit your protein and calorie numbers. Keep in mind that 1 gram (g; 0.04 ounces or 0.004 cups) of fat equals about 9 calories and that 1 g of carbohydrates equals 4 calories. You'll need carbs and fats to meet your daily calorie requirements. How you meet them is up to you. This is what makes flexible dieting fun.

Calorie Calculations

Training age, as I indicated earlier, affects your calorie intake. In the first section of this book, I introduced you to Alan Aragon's Natural Lean Muscle Mass Gain Model:

Category	Years Training	Muscle Gain
Beginner	1 or less	1–1.5% total body weight per month
Intermediate	2–3	0.5 –1% total body weight per month
Advanced	5 or more	0.25–0.5% total body weight per month

Using this model, we can calculate the calories you need daily to gain muscle. Before that, though, we need to determine your maintenance calorie intake — the amount of calories you need to eat for your body weight to stay the same.

Because you'll be training 3–6 days per week, I recommend the following calculation:

Maintenance calories = body weight (lb.) x 15

For example, if you are 150 lb. (68 kg), the calculation is

Maintenance calories = 150 x 15 = 2,250 calories per day

Knowing your maintenance calories, we can determine your muscle-building calories. To do this, we'll consult Alan Aragon's model above and bear in mind that it takes roughly 3,500 calories per week beyond your maintenance calories to gain 1 lb. (0.5 kg) of body weight.

Beginner Calories

According to Aragon, a beginner can gain up to 1.5% of total body weight a month, or up to 0.375% per week. To calculate how many extra calories beyond maintenance calories you need to eat weekly to meet Aragon's muscle mass gain estimates, use the following formula:

Weekly extra calories = body weight (lb.) x 0.00375 x 3,500 extra calories

For a 150 lb. individual, the calculation looks like this:

Weekly extra calories = 150 x 0.00375 x 3,500 = 1,968.75 extra calories per week

Now divide the result for calories per week by 7 to determine your daily extra calories:

Extra daily calories = 1,968.75 / 7 = 281 extra calories per day

To determine your total daily calories, inclusive of maintenance and extra calories, do the following calculation:

Total daily calories = maintenance calories + extra daily calories

The total calories calculation for a 150 lb. person looks like this:

Total daily calories = 2,250 + 281 = 2,531 total calories daily

Intermediate Calories

Aragon indicates that an intermediate trainee can gain up to 1% of total body weight a month, or up to 0.25% a week. Use this formula to calculate the extra calories you need per week:

Weekly extra calories = body weight (lb.) x 0.0025 x 3,500 calories

For a 150 lb. individual, the calculation is as follows:

Weekly extra calories = 150 x 0.0025 x 3,500 = 1,312.5 extra calories per week

Dividing this result by 7 gives the extra calories needed daily:

Extra daily calories = 1,312.5 / 7 = 188 extra calories per day

To determine your total daily calories, inclusive of maintenance and extra calories, do the following calculation:

Total daily calories = maintenance calories + extra daily calories

For a 150 lb. person, the total calories calculation is

Total daily calories = 2,250 + 188 = 2,438 total calories daily

Advanced Calories

An advanced trainee, by Aragon's estimates, can gain up to 0.5% of total body weight per month, or up to 0.125% a week. Calculating how many extra calories you need per week requires this formula:

Weekly extra calories = body weight (lb.) x 0.00125 x 3,500 calories

The calculation for a 150 lb. person looks like this:

Weekly extra calories = 150 x 0.00125 x 3,500 = 656.25 extra calories per week

Divide this result by 7 to get the extra calories you need daily:

Extra daily calories = 656.25 / 7 = 93.75 extra calories per day

Now determine your total daily calories, inclusive of maintenance and extra calories:

Total daily calories = maintenance calories + extra daily calories

A 150 lb. person requires the following total calories calculation:

Total daily calories = 2,250 + 93.75 = 2,344 total calories daily

What If I'm Not Gaining?

Weigh yourself weekly. If in a month you haven't gained the weight stipulated by Aragon, you will need to up your calories. Recalculate your maintenance calories using body weight x 16, instead of 15, and redo your other calculations. If another month passes without gain, recalculate your maintenance calories using body weight x 17 and redo your other calculations. Continue this process until you are gaining weight in line with Aragon's model.

You will need to redo your calculations monthly using your new body weight, as any weight gain will increase your maintenance calorie requirements. A bigger person needs more calories.

Protein Calculations

Calculating protein requirements is easy. It's unclear if what many people think, that the more protein the better, is correct, but there is clear consensus on a minimum effective daily dose of protein, at about 0.82 g/lb. of body weight. A 200 lb. (91 kg) individual needs at least 164 g (6 ounces or 0.7 cups) of protein a day. This doesn't mean that more is bad for you. Protein helps with satiety, and most people enjoy eating a lot of it.

For simplicity's sake, I recommend consuming 1 g of protein per pound of body weight daily, or 200 g (7 ounces or 0.8 cups) for a 200 lb. individual. This puts you over the minimum effective dose, so if you consume less you'll still be fine. You can, of course, also use the minimum effective dose of 0.82 g/lb. of body weight. Just don't go below the calculation for your body weight.

Here are sample calorie and protein numbers based on 1 g/lb. of body weight:

Body Weight (lb.)	Protein (g)	Calories (Beginner)	Calories (Intermediate)	Calories (Advanced)
150	150	2,531	2,438	2,344
175	175	2,953	2,844	2,734
200	200	3,375	3,250	3,125
225	225	3,797	3,656	3,516

References

Hartman, J. W., D. R. Moore, and S. M. Phillips. "Resistance Training Reduces Whole-Body Protein Turnover and Improves Net Protein Retention in Untrained Young Males." *Applied Physiology, Nutrition and Metabolism* 31 (2006): 557–64.

Hoffman J. R., N. A. Ratamess, J. Kang, M. J. Falvo, and A. D. Faigenbaum. "Effect of Protein Intake on Strength, Body Composition and Endocrine Changes in Strength/Power Athletes." *Journal of the International Society of Sports Nutrition* 3, no. 12-8 (Dec. 13, 2006).

Lemon, P. W. "Effects of Exercise on Dietary Protein Requirements." *International Journal of Sport Nutrition* 8, no. 4 (Dec. 1998): 426–47.

Lemon P. W., M. A. Tarnopolsky, J. D. Macdougall, and S. A. Atkinson. "Protein Requirements and Muscle Mass/Strength Changes during Intensive Training in Novice Bodybuilders." *Journal of Applied Physiology* 73, no. 2 (Aug. 1992): 767–75.

McCargar L. J., M. T. Clandinin, A. N. Belcastro, and K. Walker. "Dietary Carbohydrate-to-Fat Ratio: Influence on Whole-Body Nitrogen Retention, Substrate Utilization, and Hormone Response in Healthy Male Subjects." *American Journal of Clinical Nutrition* 49, no. 6 (June 1989): 1169–78.

Millward, D. J. "Macronutrient Intakes as Determinants of Dietary Protein and Amino Acid Adequacy." *Journal of Nutrition* 134, no. 6 (June 1, 2004): 1588S–1596S.

Moore, D. R., N. C. Del Bel, K. I. Nizi, J. W. Hartman, J. E. Tang, D. Armstrong, and S. M. Phillips. "Resistance Training Reduces Fasted- and Fed-State Leucine Turnover and Increases Dietary Nitrogen Retention in Previously Untrained Young Men." *Journal of Nutrition* 137 (2006): 985–91.

Phillips, S. M. and L. J. Van Loon. "Dietary Protein for Athletes: From Requirements to Optimum Adaptation." *Journal of Sports Sciences* 29, no. S1 (2011): S29–38.

Pikosky, M. A., T. J. Smith, A. Grediagin, C. Castaneda-Sceppa, L. Byerley, E. L. Glickman, and A. J. Young. "Increased Protein Maintains Nitrogen Balance during Exercise-Induced Energy Deficit." *Medicine & Science in Sports & Exercise* 40, no. 3 (March 2008): 505–12.

Rennie, M. J. and K. D. Tipton. "Protein and Amino Acid Metabolism during and after Exercise and the Effects of Nutrition." *Annual Review of Nutrition* 20 (2000): 457–83.

Rozenek, R., P. Ward, S. Long, and J. Garhammer. "Effects of High-Calorie Supplements on Body Composition and Muscular Strength Following Resistance Training." *Journal of Sports Medicine and Physical Fitness* 42, no. 3 (Sept. 2002): 340–7.

Tarnopolsky, M. A., J. D. MacDougall, and S. A. Atkinson. "Influence of Protein Intake and Training Status on Nitrogen Balance and Lean Body Mass." *Journal of Applied Physiology* 64, no. 1 (Jan. 1988): 187–93.

Walberg, J. L., M. K. Leidy, D. J. Sturgill, D. E. Hinkle, S. J. Ritchey, and D. R. Sebolt. "Macronutrient Content of a Hypoenergy Diet Affects Nitrogen Retention and Muscle Function in Weight Lifters." *International Journal of Sports Medicine* 9, no. 4 (Aug. 1988): 261–6.

Chapter 25:
Getting Lean and Mean

Building muscle is one thing, but if you want to look amazing you'll have to have muscle and low body fat levels to show off the muscle. We all know that one guy who is forever bulking. Sure, he's neither fat nor skinny, but he also doesn't look jacked. You want to look jacked.

If you've seen the television show *It's Always Sunny in Philadelphia*, you'll be familiar Mac. It was a running joke for the first six seasons that Mac was jacked. He's always bragging about working out, but he only goes to the gym occasionally and is really quite average. In season seven, Mac is transformed, bulking up with 50 lb. of pure fat. He's always eating, yet he continues acting jacked. Everyone else knows he's just fat.

Sadly, there are many people like Mac. They chase muscle. They bulk. But they're simply fat. Don't fool yourself. Strive to be muscular and lean. Make it a goal never to exceed 15–16% body fat, and you'll look good year-round and always be proud of your body.

This chapter teaches you how to be lean. It ensures that all the muscle you're diligently building gets shown off and maintained.

Three Rules for Fat Loss

Fat Loss Rule #1: Caloric Deficit

What do the following diets have in common?

- If It Fits Your Macros (IIFYM)
- Ketogenic
- Atkins
- Intermittent fasting
- Weight Watchers
- Zone
- South Beach

They shed weight by caloric deficit. Simply put, burn more calories than you eat, and you'll lose weight. A caloric deficit is attainable whether or not you diet or exercise. If you want to lose fat, you need to be in a caloric deficit. And I recommend that you start with the formula of body weight (lb.) x 12 and adjusting from there. If you're 200 lbs, eat 2,400 calories a day.

Fat Loss Rule #2: High Protein

The weight you lose through caloric deficit can be fat, muscle, or both. You want to lose fat not muscle. So you need to consume protein at a minimum of

0.82g/lb. of body weight per day. A 200 lb. person will need an absolute minimum of 164 g of protein daily.

Fat Loss Rule #3: Strength

Even the combination of high protein and caloric deficit won't guarantee fat loss. You also must maintain your muscle mass by strength training. Here's the simplest formula for fat loss: caloric deficit + high protein + strength training = fat loss.

How Fast Can I Lose Fat?

There's a maximum speed at which you can lose fat. If you diet too aggressively, you'll lose fat and muscle. This isn't good. You want to hold onto your muscle. Your goal in dieting is fat loss. And generally the fastest you can lose fat without losing muscle is when you shed about 1% of your body weight a week. I say generally because there are exceptions. You can probably lose fat quicker if you're obese, for instance. But you can't go wrong with the 1% rule.

Calories for Maximum Fat Loss

Using the 1% rule, we can calculate the calories you should eat daily to lose fat. First, though, we must determine your maintenance calorie intake—the amount of calories you need to preserve your body weight:

Maintenance calories = body weight (lb.) x 15

For a 150 lb. individual, the calculation is

Maintenance calories = 150 x 15 = 2,250 calories per day

Now that we know your maintenance calories, we can determine the calories required for you to lose weight. We know from above that you can lose 1% of your body weight per week without sacrificing muscle. We also know, from a previous chapter, that it takes roughly 3,500 calories a week beyond your maintenance calories to gain 1 lb. (0.5 kg) of body weight. It's no big step then to see that it would take a deficit of roughly 3,500 calories a week below your weekly maintenance calories to lose 1 lb. of body weight. So the following formula applies:

Calories in 1% = body weight (lb.) x 0.01 x 3,500 calories

The calculation for a 150 lb. person looks like this:

Calories in 1% = 150 x 0.01 x 3,500 calories = 5,250 calories

A 150 lb. guy seeking to lose 1% body weight a week will need to eat 5,250 calories a week less than his weekly maintenance calorie intake. Divide 5,250 calories by 7, and that guy has a 750 calorie deficit per day. Now subtract that daily deficit from your maintenance calories:

Maximum fat loss calories = maintenance – deficit

A 150 lb. individual would use the following calculation:

Maximum fat loss calories = 2,250 – 750 = 1,500 calories per day

Hate all that math? Just multiply your body weight, in pounds, by 10, and, voila, you have your maximum fat-loss calories. See the following examples.

Maximum Fat-Loss Cheat Sheet

	Formula	If 150 lb.	If 200 lb.	If 250 lb.
Calories (kcal)	Body weight (lb.) x 10	1,500 per day	2,000 per day	2,500 per day
Minimum Protein (g)	Body weight (lb.) x 0.82	123 g	164 g	205 g

Chapter 26:
Nutrient timing: Is it worth it?

The beauty of flexible dieting is that you can eat what you want, when you want. Nutrient timing dictates that you eat your proteins, carbohydrates, and fats at certain times of the day and based on how much you're exercising. Is nutrient timing worth the loss of flexibility?

The Anabolic Window

When I was in university, the belief was that you had an anabolic window of about 30–90 minutes post-workout to consume the carbohydrates and proteins needed to recover and to build muscle. As soon as my last weight hit the floor, I'd race home to eat plain chicken breast and rice. If someone got in my way, I'd rage. There was no way I was missing that window.

This was a stressor. It increased my levels of cortisol, a hormone that in high levels leads to fat gain and a compromised immune system. The goal of my workouts was to build muscle and lose fat. Yet my high levels of cortisol made both difficult. I couldn't lose weight or stay lean, and I was sick frequently and forced to take time off training. The anabolic window did me more harm than good.

Evolution of the Science

In 2004, Drs. John Ivy and Robert Portman published *Nutrient Timing: The Future of Sports Nutrition*, at the time a game-changing book for the health and fitness communities. Using then state-of-the-art science, the authors appeared to prove the anabolic window and the benefit of consuming carbohydrates and proteins within 30–90 minutes after a workout.

The problem was, their studies were short not long term and looked only at protein synthesis and glycogen replenishment, which was great at the time. But the studies failed to ask, Did meeting the anabolic window work better for fat loss, muscle gain, and strength gains? The answer is "no." But it also doesn't hinder the trainee, unless the trainee gets stressed trying to make the window, like yours truly.

What I Do

Ultimately, diet comes down to personal preference. If you want flexibility, eat what you want, when you want it. The only caveat is that you eat within 5% of your macros every day.

My preference is a light nutrient timing approach. This is less about body composition than about how certain foods make me feel. I've found, for example, that eating carbs early in the day makes me sleepy, less focused, almost sloth like. This is detrimental on workdays. So I don't eat carbs until after work. I've found this to be the case with many clients and colleagues.

I've also discovered that if I eat carbs leading up to and following my workout, I don't feel sloth like. The exercise helps take away the drowsiness. My hypothesis is that this is due to the short-term effects of nutrient timing, involving protein synthesis and glycogen replenishment. I've also found that consuming carbohydrates during my workout enables me to handle increased sets and reps. This, obviously, is beneficial for building muscle. So I eat carbs before, during, and after most of my workouts.

I also eat carbs for my final meal of the day in preparation for bed. The carbs help me relax and fall asleep. I believe that sleep is the most important thing to optimize if you want to change your body composition. So I take it seriously and do what I can to ensure I get it.

Your Nutrient Timing Plan of Action

Your priority with your diet is to hit your macros consistently every day. Be as flexible with your diet as you want, just make sure that you hit your macros.

Once you can do this consistently for two weeks, I recommend experimenting with nutrient timing.

Try eating carbohydrates as part of your last meal of the day to see if this improves your sleep. Also try not eating carbs until you are finished work, unless you eat them around your workout. See how this makes you feel. Were you more focused and productive? If so, keep doing it. Did it have the opposite effect and make you feel terrible? Then stop. This is science at its most basic. Experiment, and if it works, keep doing it. If not, don't do it.

Reference

Ivy, John, and Robert Portman. *Nutrient Timing: The Future of Sports Nutrition*. Laguna Beach, CA: Basic Health Publications, 2004.

Chapter 27:
Supplements: What SUPP Man?

"Hey bro, what "pre-workout" are you taking?" Walk into any gym, and you'll inevitably hear someone talk about their "pre-workout." Generally, this means they ingested a high-stimulant supplement before their workout to amp them up and give them energy.

I knew a guy who was addicted to buying the latest and greatest supplements. I'm willing to bet he tried 70–80% of the pre-workout supplements on the market between 2007 and 2013. He fell for the marketing and the hype. He also fell for weight gainers, fat burners, multivitamins, protein powders, and every gel, drink, or powder under the sun. If a supplement was endorsed by an athlete or celebrity, he tried it. By the end of 2013, he admitted to spending over $28,000 on supplements. The only thing those fat burners did was burn a giant hole in his wallet.

You're reading this chapter because you care about your body. You want to take a few supplements. That's fine. The right supplements work and work well. Know, however, that you can get fantastic results without supplements. The classic, drug-free bodybuilders of the 1960s and 70s had access to few supplements and built great bodies.

Before taking supplements, look at your lifestyle. If your diet is poor, if you're skipping workouts, and if you're not getting enough sleep, supplements should not be your priority. Master your diet, workouts, and sleep and then revisit this chapter. Master the basics and then optimize with supplements.

Ingredients Matter

Your local supplement store will bombard you with marketing in an effort to make money. Don't be fooled by the hype. Look beyond it at what matters: the ingredients. Many supplements in your local shop are light on ingredients. If you want the best bang for your buck, I suggest buying online in bulk pure-form supplements, or as close as possible. This is safer; you'll know what you're getting.

Below, I list supplements that I've found effective or that are proven effective. I've categorized them according to when they should be taken. These are just suggestions; I'm not a doctor, so please consult one before trying anything from this list.

Anytime

Fish oil. Studies show that fish oil—and we're not talking cod liver oil—reduces triglycerides, helps with depression, decreases anxiety, and provides cardiovascular benefits. Buy high omega-3 fish oil in liquid form and follow the dosage on the bottle. (If you eat oily fish several times a week, you don't need to supplement with fish oil.)

Vitamin D3. Unless you're a surfer or an outdoor worker, your vitamin D levels are probably low. Have your doctor verify. Vitamin D keeps your bones strong and healthy, boosts testosterone, and is an essential vitamin. Most people require only 1,000 IU per day. But people who get no sunlight will need higher dosages. On dark days in winter, I take upward of 5,000 IU.

Whey isolate. This is my favorite form of protein powder. It's cheap; easy to digest (for most people); and a simple way to supplement your protein intake. Whey isolate powder is high in protein and will help you hit your daily protein targets. Buy a supplement that is over 90% whey isolate by weight to ensure that you're getting little filler and mostly ingredient.

Creatine monohydrate. Research reveals that creatine helps build strength, muscle, and power and is entirely safe. It makes a big difference in the gym. I take creatine monohydrate daily. Men should take 5 g (1 teaspoon) a day, and women should take 2.5 g (1/2 teaspoon) a day.

Beta-alanine. Beta-alanine buffers lactic acid and promotes muscle healing, recovery, and contractions. It'll help you run longer, play harder, lift more reps, and recover faster. Whereas creatine helps you lift more weight, beta-alanine helps you lift more reps. Combining the two will dramatically improve your workouts. Preliminary research shows best results with two 3.2 g (1 teaspoon) dosages daily, one in the morning, one in the afternoon. Warning: beta-alanine gives a temporary pins-and-needles feeling the first couple of weeks.

Pre-workout

Caffeine. Technically, caffeine is a drug, a substance other than food that can affect your mind or body. Caffeine boosts energy 10–15 minutes after ingestion. I find 100–200 mg of caffeine in pill form works best before a workout, not every workout, just especially hard ones.

The Muscle Cocktail

The following is heavily based on bro-science and my experimentation and is heavily influenced by the practice of professional bodybuilder John Meadows.

Pre-workout Muscle Cocktail

Some 30–60 minutes before my workouts, I ingest the following:

- ½ cup of oats (dry measured)
- 40 g of protein as whey isolate
- 2 tsp of butter

The goal is a sustained release of carbohydrates and amino acids into the bloodstream to aid endurance and help shuttle amino acids into muscle cells. Studies are insufficient to prove or disprove this, but this blend does help me with energy and building muscle. And it's a delicious meal that gets me "in the game" before a tough workout. I wouldn't recommend eating this before a morning workout unless you are very hungry and must eat before going to the gym.

Workout Muscle Cocktail

During workout set breaks, I like to sip on a drink of the following:

- 20–40 g of hydrolyzed whey protein
- 40–80 g of highly branched cyclic dextrin

Hydrolyzed whey protein is quickly digested and broken down and enters your bloodstream rapidly. Highly branched cyclic dextrin is a quickly digested carbohydrate that readily breaks down and enters your bloodstream rapidly. Ingested together during workouts, they increase endurance, helping you complete more reps and, ultimately, build more muscle, and help shuttle glucose and amino acids into your muscle cells. This, too, hasn't been proven or disproven, so experiment. I and many of my clients enjoy the benefits.

Remember to count you pre-workout and workout muscle cocktails among your daily macros. During a fat-loss phase, when your calories are low, these cocktails could account for 50-90% of your total calories. In this case, you should skip the cocktails in favor of real foods.

Supplements are optional. As worthwhile as it may be to experiment, your focus must be on working out consistently, giving it your all in the gym, hitting your macros constantly, and getting at least seven hours of deep sleep a night. This yields results.

References

Bischoff-Ferrari, Heike A., Walter C. Willett, John B. Wong, Andreas E. Stuck, Hannes B. Staehelin, E. John Orav, Anna Thoma, Douglas P. Kiel, and Jana Henschkowski. "Prevention of Nonvertebral Fractures with Oral Vitamin D and Dose Dependency." *Archives of Internal Medicine* 169, no. 6 (2009): 551.

Candow, Darren G., Philip D. Chilibeck, Darren G. Burke, Kristie D. Mueller, and Jessica D. Lewis. "Effect of Different Frequencies of Creatine Supplementation on Muscle Size and Strength in Young Adults." *Journal of Strength and Conditioning Research* 25, no. 7 (2011): 1831–838.

Favero, Serena del, Hamilton Roschel, Guilherme Artioli, Carlos Ugrinowitsch, Valmor Tricoli, André Costa, Renato Barroso, Ana Lua Negrelli, Maria Concepción Otaduy, Cláudia da Costa Leite, Antonio Herbert Lancha-Junior, and Bruno Gualano. "Creatine but Not Betaine Supplementation Increases Muscle Phosphorylcreatine Content and Strength Performance." *Amino Acids* 42, no. 6 (2011): 2299–305.

Hobson, R. M., B. Saunders, G. Ball, R. C. Harris, and C. Sale. "Effects of Beta-alanine Supplementation on Exercise Performance: A Meta-analysis." *Amino Acids* 43, no. 1 (2012): 25–37.

Kiecolt-Glaser, Janice K., Martha A. Belury, Rebecca Andridge, William B. Malarkey, and Ronald Glaser. "Omega-3 Supplementation Lowers Inflammation and Anxiety in Medical Students: A Randomized Controlled Trial." *Brain, Behavior, and Immunity* 25, no. 8 (2011): 1725–734.

Seftel, Allen. "Re: Effect of Vitamin D Supplementation on Testosterone Levels in Men." *Journal of Urology* 186, no. 1 (2011): 239–40.

Sublette, M. Elizabeth, Steven P. Ellis, Amy L. Geant, and J. John Mann. "Meta-Analysis of the Effects of Eicosapentaenoic Acid (EPA) in Clinical Trials in Depression." *Journal of Clinical Psychiatry* 72, no. 12 (2011): 1577–584.

Toth, P. P. "Dose-response Effects of Omega-3 Fatty Acids on Triglycerides, Inflammation, and Endothelial Function in Healthy Persons with Moderate Hypertriglyceridemia." *Yearbook of Endocrinology* (2011): 51–54.

Chapter 28:
The Lean Bulk Cycle

When you start training, you'll feel as if every calorie needs to go to building muscle, especially if you're skinny. I was constantly overeating when I began training seriously. I had no idea what I was doing. I just picked a calorie count out of the air and ran with it: 3,000 calories a day split evenly at 33.3% for each of proteins, carbohydrates, and fats. This was approximately 250 g of protein, 250 g of carbohydrates, and 111 g of fats per day.

I was 19, just starting university, and weighed approximately 155 lb. In three months, I gained approximately 27 lb. of muscle. I should only have been eating about 2,600–2700 calories a day and gaining 1 lb. per week. So I was overeating by 300 calories a day. I was also drinking heavily two nights a week, the equivalent of nearly 20 drinks a week, which is classified as excessive.

Whenever I drank, I could eat huge amounts and was known as the "human garbage disposal." I once recorded what I ate on a night of drinking. In two hours, I ate 7,000 calories in addition to the 3,000 I'd already eaten that day, for 10,000 calories in one day!

Yet I still gained 27 lb. of muscle in a short period of time. I'm 28 years old, and to attempt the same dietary habits would probably push me to a nearly obese 250 lb. Why could I overeat at 19 and build a lean body? Why can't I do that now? Age, obviously, has a bit to do with it, but it's more because I was a beginner. In gym talk, I benefited from newbie gains.

After my first year of training, I couldn't continue the same lifestyle. The honeymoon with newbie gains was over, and I was gaining fat fast. I knew it was time to do something when I reached 200 lb. and 20% body fat. I adopted a strict, low-carb, low-calorie diet and lost 9.5% body fat and 21 lb. in only 10 weeks, referred to as cutting. But I hated my life. I was a hermit. I'd say no when my friends invited me out. I didn't want to be the depressed guy sipping water while his buddies had the time of their lives.

After 10 weeks of misery, I upped my calories and noticed that I was gaining muscle and strength at an accelerated rate while staying lean. I was diligent with my body fat measurements, and I noticed that once I got above 13–14% my gains would stall and it seemed easier to gain fat than muscle; the opposite of what I wanted. So I'd resume dieting to lower my body fat to 10–11%. At that level, I found it was easier to resume gaining muscle while staying lean. I'd bulk up again until my gains would stall, and then I'd diet down.

The cycle continued, and the lean bulk cycle was born. I've found that it's easier to gain muscle if you are lean.

Most guys make the same mistake I did when I started training: bulk up and get fat and then cut down. What happens is you only look good for a few weeks a year, near the end of your cut. The rest of the year you are chubby and bulky. It's not logical. You work out to look good and feel good. Why go on long bulks and cuts to look good only a couple of weeks a year? It makes no sense, but everyone seems to do it.

Bulk up to 13-14% body fat, and you will still have visible abs. You'll still look and feel great. And you'll find it easy to gain muscle while you're lean. Once you've exhausted your newbie gains, the lean bulk cycle is the way to go.

How to Do the Lean Bulk Cycle

Bulk up to 13–14% body fat. Then cut down to 8–11%. Repeat the process of bulking and cutting between 8–14% body fat until you've attained your perfect body.

Workouts. Use the workouts given in this book; they stay the same whether you are bulking or cutting. The goal of a workout is to build muscle and strength, not burn calories. Your diet dictates whether you gain or lose weight.

Diet. When cutting, use the calorie and macronutrient calculations from the fat-loss chapter. When bulking, use the calorie and macronutrient calculations for muscle gain.

What to Expect. Depending on your body fat levels, the two phases of the lean bulk cycle—cutting and bulking—can last anywhere between 4–12 weeks each. This means you will constantly be doing a mini bulk or a mini cut. The good news is that you will always be either at or below 13–14% body fat and will always look great. You will also always be gaining muscle and strength.

If you're above 14% body fat. Use the dieting recommendations in the fat loss chapter until you are within the 8–14% body fat range. This puts you within lean bulk cycle body fat levels, and you can pick up from there, cutting or bulking as required.

Bulk or cut. Measure your body fat percentage with either the InBody 520 or BodyMetrix Ultrasound wand. Your local gym might carry this equipment and allow you to use it. After the measurement, decide. Are you 14% body fat or over? You need to cut. Are you 10% body fat? It's up to you if you want to get leaner or if you want to bulk. Either way, you need to earn your right to bulk. This means you need to be lean first.

SECTION 4:
LIVE AN AWESOME LIFE

Chapter 29:
How to Be Happy

You want to be happy with your body because you want to be a happy person. Don't assume, however, that merely developing a fantastic body will make you happy.

Happiness comes from the inside. Changing your physical appearance will help, but it's not the end all and be all. If you added 30 lb. of muscle to your skinny frame, yes, you'd probably be happy. But would you be happier yet if you shredded that 30 lb. of muscle and maintained your body fat at below 10%? Maybe, maybe not.

You might have problems in your life. Maybe you hate your job or you are struggling financially. Maybe you're single and want a family. Maybe you're married but hate your significant other. These are all problems that can be fixed. You just need to look deep within and find the things that make you happy and do more of them. You also need to find the things that sabotage your happiness and get rid of them.

Sometimes, building the perfect body sacrifices our happiness. When I was 21 years old, I strove for sub

10% body fat. I was on an extreme diet and could only eat meat and vegetables. I stopped going out with friends and doing anything social that involved food. My life sucked. This, of course, was before I discovered flexible dieting and the lean bulk cycle. But even then, achieving extreme goals may call for sacrifices.

This is why you need to find a sweet spot. You need to build a physique that you are happy with while ensuring that you are not making a ton of sacrifices and are still able to be social. You need, in other words, to find the happy medium between the sacrifices and inflexibility required to build the perfect body and to hit your macros 100% of the time and eating like a slob and not training and having a disgusting body.

Analyze your body on a scale of 1 to 10, with 10 being absolute perfection and 1 being disgusting, and find a number where your body image happiness is sufficiently high that you'd feel good in a bathing suit yet confident enough to enjoy social events without guilt. My body happiness is between 8 and 9. I can still go out with friends, eat a lot of great food, and have a few drinks. But I also track my macros and train four times a week. This gives me an overall life happiness of 9.5–10. And that's what counts.

Make sacrifices at the start of your training. You'll need to if your body image happiness is 3, for example. But once you reach a body image happiness of 8–9, relax and maintain.

At every stage of your training, increase your body image happiness by doing one thing that doesn't involve working out or dieting: learn to love yourself. Free yourself of negative relationships, forgive people who caused you trauma, meditate. This is not nonsense. Love yourself, and your overall happiness will soar.

Building a great body—without undue sacrifice—is the perfect first step toward loving yourself. And this book gives you all the tools you need to build a body that you can be proud of and happy with. It all starts with muscle.

Chapter 30:
Closing Thoughts

You now have the blueprint to building the body of your dreams and achieving happiness. It doesn't matter if you're a beginner, intermediate, or advanced trainee, you will benefit from this book.

If someone had told me when I was 19 that I would write a book on building muscle, I would have laughed. That skinny-fat guy with zero confidence is a much different person today, and it's all because of everything I've learned about fitness.

Fitness changed my life. It's my passion. It's my career. Transform your body, and you transform your mindset. You realize that making changes in your life isn't that hard. It gave me the confidence I needed to meet girls and get a girlfriend. It gave me the confidence to take the difficult path and become a personal trainer instead of a rocket scientist. It gave me the confidence to travel the world for three years and to build JMax Fitness into what it is today.

Gaining muscle was the greatest thing I ever could have done for my life. I hope that you'll feel the same way.